W9-AKX-382

Lifting the Veil of
Menopause

Charlene,
  1 hope you find this book
informative and easy to
read.
Long time no see ☺
1 wish you the best in the
coming year
    Sincerely
      N. Tuakli
        2015

Lifting the Veil of *Menopause*

A Natural Solution

Nadu A. Tuakli, MD, MPH

Copyright © 2015 by Nadu A. Tuakli, MD, MPH.

Library of Congress Control Number:		2015907299
ISBN:	Hardcover	978-1-5035-6883-9
	Softcover	978-1-5035-6884-6
	eBook	978-1-5035-6885-3

All rights reserved. No part of this book may be reproduced or transmitted in any form or by any means, electronic or mechanical, including photocopying, recording, or by any information storage and retrieval system, without permission in writing from the copyright owner.

This book is intended solely for informational and educational purposes and not as personal advice for any individual. All efforts have been made to assure the accuracy of the information contained in this book as of the date of publication.

Suggestions in this book are not meant to substitute for medical evaluation and recommendations by your physician.

All matters regarding health care require medical supervision. The author and publisher are not liable for any loss, injury, or damage allegedly arising from any information or suggestion in this book.

Print information available on the last page.

Rev. date: 06/18/2015

To order additional copies of this book, contact:
Xlibris
1-888-795-4274
www.Xlibris.com
Orders@Xlibris.com
636420

Contents

Abbreviations

HRT	hormone-replacement therapy
BHRT	bioidentical hormone therapy
WHO	World Health Organization
GYN	gynecology or gynecologist
BRCA	A gene that is found in families with a high incidence of ovarian and breast cancer
NIH	National Institutes of Health in Bethesda. A government research institution
BPPV	benign paroxysmal vertigo, a condition of unknown cause that causes dizziness and lightheadedness
NHLBI	A branch of the NIH
WHI	Women's Health Initiative, a study done by the NHI to see the effects of hormone therapy
OCP	Oral Contraceptive Pill
FSH	Follicle Stimulating Hormone
LH	Luteinizing Hormone
PMS	Premenstrual Syndrome
BMI	Body Mass Index a weight to height ratio used as an indicator of obesity
TAHBSO	A hysterectomy where the uterus, tubes and ovaries are removed
FDA	Food and Drug Administration
DHEA	Dehydroepiandrosterone a steroid hormone
SSRI	Class of antidepressant medications that increase serotonin in the brain
MS	Multiple Sclerosis

ED	Erectile Dysfunction
RCOG	Royal College of Obstetricians and Gynecologists (UK)
E1	Estrone
E2	Estradiol
E3	Estriol
P/E	Ratio between Progesterone and Estrogen

Introduction

*Health is a state of complete physical, mental, and social
well-being, and not merely the absence of disease or infirmity.*
—World Health Organization (WHO)[1]

I AM PROUD OF the practical wisdom I have acquired during the last thirty years of practicing medicine. I learned a lot in medical school and then at places like Harvard and Johns Hopkins, but this kind of wisdom is not taught in school. It is the wisdom of experience that allows doctors to polish their art. It has fueled my desire to want to continue to make a difference in my patients' lives, particularly in the area of women's health and longevity. Over the years I have had the opportunity to treat a lot of menopausal patients and have seen firsthand the dilemmas it can create.

In addition to my clinical practice I have always enjoyed teaching, whether currently as an assistant professor at Georgetown Medical School or under less official hats like preceptor for nurse-practitioner students from Duke, Maryland, and Marymount universities or just as a mentor for high school seniors. Most important, I love to teach my patients. This is my most important role as a doctor and the reason I've written this book.

How often have you heard the old saying "knowledge is power"? Never is that more true than for a patient. Often I find that even though I am an experienced physician, many of my colleagues are unwilling

---

[1] Preamble to the Constitution of the World Health Organization as adopted by the International Health Conference, New York, June 19–22, 1946; signed on July 22, 1946, by the representatives of sixty-one states (Official Records of the World Health Organization, no. 2, p. 100) and entered into force on April 7, 1948.

to engage in a meaningful debate about hormones with me, much less with an inquisitive patient.

My main goal in writing this book is to give readers the best medical advice I can about menopause and its symptoms, and to show how women who are suffering from symptoms can improve them through various therapies—particularly hormone balancing. Having this information will allow you to discuss the subject knowledgeably with your doctor. My take on this particular subject is different from what you may have heard from other doctors or read in the mainstream media, and later in the book I will explain why I say this.

I want to spread the word about bioidentical hormones as a viable and likely healthier treatment option in an area of women's health that has been neglected, dismissed, underreported, and misunderstood for decades.

For centuries women have accepted that menopause signals the end of a woman's vitality and desirability, with an inevitable decrease in her quality of life. It's time to tell the truth! A woman's quality of life, including her sex life, can continue throughout her lifespan, which, at menopause, is only halfway, after all. An excellent quality of life is available to any woman who wants it. Depending on where you live, it may be a little challenging to find a doctor who will help, but when you do, it will be well worthwhile.

I find the lack of knowledge regarding hormonal issues in menopausal women to be staggering, and as the years go by I see it doesn't get any better. In my view, many women suffer needlessly from the sheer lack of valid and reliable scientific information. I am determined to help.

Menopause is often the elephant in the room; the woman going through it and her family members may feel uncomfortable talking about it. Sometimes the whole concept can be hard to explain and even harder to understand.

As one patient told me, "My husband just doesn't get it." She tried to explain to him that she thought she had a hormonal problem, but he felt that she was just overly stressed.

"My mother went through menopause without any problems," her husband says. (*Really? he discussed that with his mother?* I thought skeptically). Most people decide to not discuss it.

On the other hand, when menopause *is* talked about, it's often with old-fashioned ideas in mind. Well-meaning loved ones will try to convince a professional woman to cut back on her professional activities—a problem *men* don't seem to have. Somehow I don't think that kind of advice would fly if she were First Lady or head of the Reserve Bank.

This pertains especially when women are making huge strides professionally. Here in the states we have already had women as presidential candidates, and many countries have female heads of state. It is inconceivable that women like these, with so much responsibility, would not have their menopausal symptoms handled efficiently, or worse yet, be overmedicated with drugs.

Having lived and worked professionally all over the world, I am very much aware of the different cultural attitudes toward women and menopause. Although they are gradually changing, none are particularly progressive.

My passion regarding menopause began around twenty years ago with Mandy (see Mandy's story a few pages ahead), whose plight so galvanized me that I began to research hormone-replacement therapy (HRT) and regularly attend conferences on the topic to stay up on the latest scientific information and to compare notes and experiences with like-minded physicians.

Every week a woman comes to my office in a state of emotional crisis because her "hormones are out of whack." These women are invariably successful, up-to-date on the latest technology, and often find me after scouring the Internet looking for solutions.

They find themselves blindsided, floored, and totally out of control when they hit menopause. Their discourse ranges from "I wish I had known" to loudly demanding "Why doesn't anyone tell you this stuff?"

I believe this book addresses these issues.

Today many people get their health education from infomercials that pass for news shows, or sound bites that are driven more to entertain than to genuinely inform. It is as if health news is imitating Hollywood, delivering so-called medical information that is driven more by sensationalism and commercial interests. Unfortunately, the topic of menopause does not much lend itself to sensationalism and so is often ignored.

That is where this book comes in. Here is the information you need.

Warning: before you allow your doctor to refer you to a psychiatrist or hand you pills for anxiety and sleep, read this book.

With such a strong focus on youth, women are loath to admit they are actually menopausal because it seems to be an admission that they are in fact over the hill. The booming industry of the vainglorious and antiaging has resulted in the desire to maintain youth. However, searching for eternal youth doesn't seem to make sense when we ignore something as basic as hormone deficiency. In terms of the aging process, there are many things that you can do, but none will be more helpful for maintaining a vibrant midlife passage than managing your hormones.

The role of consumerism and market-driven economies has led to pharmaceutical companies deciding what is best for women instead of women owning their own decisions with the positive assistance of their doctors.

One of the goals of this book is to lift the veil of confusion about menopause and the use of hormones, dispel the myths that surround it, and hopefully reduce the fear and shame that so many women seem to feel about the notion of "the change."

Prevailing myths and attitudes create so much suffering, and statements like, "Menopause is a natural phenomenon—suck it up!" result in countless women feeling insecure and inadequate because despite their best efforts they *can't* "just deal with it."

In addition to dispelling these myths, I will explain how bioidentical hormone-replacement therapy (BHRT) can be used to help ease the symptoms of menopause and improve the quality of life for millions of women. No woman needs to live with untreated menopausal symptoms unless she chooses to.

Based on my experience treating thousands of women (and hundreds for menopausal symptoms), there is no doubt in my mind that bioidentical hormone-replacement therapy (BHRT) is a powerful tool—one that is underutilized because people are unnecessarily afraid of it. Too many women end up denying themselves the benefits of treatment just out of the fear that is created by a of lack of reliable information.

Bioidentical hormones are a wonderful solution for millions of women, and for the vast majority, there's no reason why they cannot take them.

Anything one takes, including hormones, drugs, and many herbs, have side effects. However, your body recognizes the molecular structure of BHRT as something it used to make, while synthetic hormones are seen by your body as foreign material. Hormones are not a panacea, but they can help you remake your life and let you get back to feeling good with a positive outlook on your future aging.

It's not about vanity. Nor is it about taking a pill that will make you aroused all the time. Most women just want to feel like themselves. In fact, the commonest complaint I get from newly menopausal women is, "I just want to feel like me."

This book was written as an educational overview for both men and women. I have tried to explain hormones in simple terms without too much science and medical language. I will discuss the mainstream scientific community's current views on bioidentical hormones, and I will say specifically why and how I believe those views may be mistaken. Finally, I will identify who is a candidate for BHRT and who is not. You should always start any treatment in consultation with your doctor, of course—but before visiting the doctor, your first duty is to educate yourself so you know what questions to ask.

The book is dotted with true stories of real patients and the challenges they have faced. We discover women who have managed to throw off their fear and confusion and seek help.

Ten thousand Americans turn fifty daily, to the tune of 3,650,000 per year. This is the baby-boomer generation that wants and demands real answers regarding their health. They will spend almost half of their lifespan after menopause and don't have the time or inclination to wilt away.

Let's create a new vision of our health that looks beyond assumptions and the obvious. A vision that challenges the discourse and envisages new possibilities for a woman's future. This vision requires that we be informed about how our bodies really work and what they need without creating false ideals and unrealistic expectations.

Please keep an open mind and process the information presented here objectively, without falling prey to the preconceived bias that has been instilled by old wives' tales, rumor-mongers, and the medical profession for generations.

To live without the benefit of this important information is foolhardy and results in a constant desire for the newest health fad or latest gimmick. I want to help create a different future for myself and other menopausal women based on truth and real information. I hope this book will lift the veil and show women their options. Read it and decide what is best for you. As you will see, one size does *not* fit all.

I hope that by the time you've reached the end of this book, you'll know much more about menopause and about the therapies that can help ease its symptoms. And just as importantly, you'll know that aging women do not need to be miserable or settle for mediocrity in terms of well-being and fulfillment.

They can feel really good as they live their healthy, vibrant lives.

Menopause is just halfway. The best is yet to come!

NADU A. TUAKLI, MD, MPH

Chapter 1

Is Fear Holding you Back?

There is nothing to fear but fear itself.
—Franklin Delano Roosevelt

A S THE BRAVE physicist and chemist Marie Curie said, "Nothing in life is to be feared, it is only to be understood."

The number-one reason my patients tell me they haven't explored options for treatment of their menopausal symptoms is that they fear the side effects and risks of taking hormones. Many women are afraid of getting cancer. Some people are just suspicious of medications, and some don't like putting anything additional into their systems, but for most women, it is about risks—potential or perceived. Most still need information to be clear about how risks are understood. Women may say they're not afraid, just cautious, but for those people who are truly afraid, this chapter is for you.

I find that it helps to talk about fear generally and specifically, so let's define our terms. Fear is defined in *Webster's Dictionary* as a feeling of uneasiness, apprehension, or concern; it's also identified as anxiety and agitation that is felt in the presence of danger. I have heard patients describe all of these feelings when talking about menopause and hormones.

There are so many fears, including fear of the unknown, fear of rebelling against society's expectations, and fear of seeking treatment, which also involves asking for help.

Let's think about where fear comes from and how it may affect us. When it comes to health, I suggest that perhaps we worry about the human condition as a whole. There is the fear of getting sick, suffering pain, getting old, decaying, declining, and ultimately the fear of death.

In addition to the big fear (of death), we can experience other types of fear, even fear of *good* things, like success. The problem comes when we allow this fear to hold us in its grip; we hold ourselves back from accomplishing what we might otherwise achieve. Fear of making a mistake is a first cousin to the fear of success. It stops us from exploring our most creative aspirations. Such fears are thought to be more typical of women than men. For example, this kind of fear stops girls from going to engineering school.

What Does this Have to Do with Taking Hormones?

Fear can create a sort of paralysis where some women become their own worst enemy. Fear about future occurrences can cause us to limit the quality of our lives in case of what might happen.

I don't think women fear hormones because they are afraid of feeling good, but there is a degree of thinking, *I don't feel* that *bad, and how do I know the side effects of the hormones won't be worse?*

Why and How Did We become Afraid of Hormones?

When it comes to hormones, our fears are exacerbated by rumors (read about the Women's Health Initiative study in chapter 7). The good news is that fear can be overcome by information and health education. The key is in understanding how your body works and what it needs. It is an amazing machine! By doing so, you can improve your daily life.

In this book I want to do the same thing that I do when I consult with patients, and that is to focus on quality of life and ease ungrounded fears by demystifying the whole concept of hormones, natural and synthetic. I tell my patients they may be surprised by what they learn if they put aside their fear for a few moments and look at the science—not the bandwagon rumors and fear-mongering but the actual science of menopause.

Hormones really aren't scary. They are just a tool in the box or the armamentarium that we have in order to achieve optimum well-being.

I'm not suggesting everyone necessarily needs to take hormones after menopause, but I do believe there are many women who would benefit from hormone therapy, yet they deny themselves that benefit out of unwarranted fear and misconceptions.

What Are You Really Afraid of?

It can help to ask yourself that question, especially when you're feeling conflicted about your menopausal symptoms. Are you afraid of relieving your menopause? Do you fear a potential side effect, or actual problems? This unexamined, amorphous fear is why so many women choose to ignore menopause until it ambushes them. If you read about the symptoms in chapter 4, you will see why I would be more scared of the symptoms than the treatment.

A lot of people, for reasons they often cannot clearly articulate, are very concerned about the idea of taking hormones. Sometimes it's just a generic fear, even though they intuitively understand the concept, for example, of supplementing thyroid hormone if their thyroid is underactive or taking insulin if they are diabetic. The prevailing wisdom is that one has to be "sick enough" to deserve to take hormones, yet even the World Health Organization (WHO) points out that health is not just about the absence of infirmity.

Some women tell me they are *glad* their hot flashes were so bad that they needed hormones because taking them made them feel better in so many other ways that improved their self-esteem and gave them a feeling of being in better control of their health.

Many of the fears women and doctors have about taking hormones are related to the side effects of birth-control pills, such as an increased incidence of blood clots. If you want to be afraid of taking hormones, be afraid of birth-control pills. Bioidentical estrogen, when used as a cream bypasses the stomach (i.e., not taken orally) and does *not* increase the risk of blood clots. [2]

Many critics of bioidentical hormone-replacement therapy (BHRT) have no qualms about women taking inordinate amounts of birth-control pills, which bear no resemblance to what the human body makes itself. Millions of young women swallow these pills every single day without concern. Society considers them an unavoidable evil, but they are more harmful than bioidentical hormones. If only there were such a thing as a bioidentical birth-control pill!

I never hear anyone ask, "Are they natural?" when talking about birth control pills. In spite of this, there is an irrational *lack* of fear with these drugs. Clearly "Big Pharma" (the term often used when referring to the giant conglomerate the pharmaceutical industry has become) does a good job of advertising and of convincing doctors and patients of their "safety," so we foolishly don't question the "wisdom" of taking them.

Some women start birth-control pills in their early twenties and continue until their mid-fifties. Young people are fearless, and they feel invincible, so they seem carefree about taking these daily doses of hormones that carry *known* risks. To me, our reactions seem backward— it would seem more rational to fear the synthetic hormones of the birth-control pills than of bioidentical hormones, which, incidentally, are used in relatively smaller doses than birth-control hormones and are not swallowed. (See chapter 6 for why it is safer not to swallow hormones.)

To make matters worse, many women are now being offered the birth-control pill when they first become perimenopausal to control symptoms caused by the hormone deficiency, such as heavy, irregular bleeding—this in spite of the fact that the birth-control package inserts clearly advise women not to take birth-control pills beyond age forty-five unless there are *compelling* reasons.

Also, many patients fearlessly take an antidepressant for menopausal symptoms but get totally freaked out at the idea of taking a hormone that their body naturally makes. Guess what? Ovaries don't make Prozac, but that drug doesn't stir up the same level of fear as the thought of hormone therapy. Did you know bioidentical hormones are made from yams?

In my experience, the fear of taking medication is also gender influenced. In stark contrast to post-menopausal women, men have no qualms about taking testosterone. Most of them come in asking to be tested "to see if I need it." They are clearly onboard with the idea of replacing what they may be missing.

It's no surprise there is some sexism at work in terms of insurance reimbursement. Erectile dysfunction in men is considered a medical problem, and medications to treat it are deemed medically necessary, so these are reimbursed by the insurance companies. But these same companies refuse to pay for compounded hormones. See the letter on page 12 sent from a pharmacy on behalf of the insurance company "Compounded Medication Alert", do you see the fear-mongering in it? The drug company lobby ensures this unfair policy toward coverage and reimbursement continues.

Fear of Change and Societal Notions

Cultural attitudes toward menopause and women in general generate fear of change, of upsetting the apple cart, and this creates fear of discovery. These cultural attitudes and assumptions go a long way towards oppressing women's desire to feel better.

The irony of this is that marketing and the media scream at all of us to be alive, feel young. Be trim, fit, and energized. Yet there is no word about doing this during menopause. The commercial community acts as if most menopausal women have simply fallen off the radar; they are invisible. Some women act accordingly.

A Doctor's Quandary

Even doctors are conflicted, so the layperson's fear is certainly understandable. Here is an example of a woman who tackled her fear by searching for information and becoming knowledgeable.

A colleague of mine, Jen, was bewildered by the whole idea of hormone replacement. A board-certified gynecologist in private practice for more than twenty years, her quandary was whether to take hormones. Her husband was an oncologist, so he saw cancer coming around every corner. When she took the hormones, he would make her feel like she was risking her life. So she would stop them and then start them again when she felt bad. She confided in me: "I really believe the women I see who are taking hormones look a lot younger, feel better, and seem to have fewer problems than those who don't." She said she realized women on HRT also maintain their weight better and are more energized. On the other hand, her husband the oncologist was constantly reminding her that she might be increasing her risk of breast cancer, even with bioidenticals.

"Like every other woman I worry about bad things like cancer," she said. So after doing a lot more research she finally went back on her hormones and started exercising. She said, "If HRT can increase my cancer risk by 0.5 percent and exercise can decrease it by 30 to 40 percent, I am happy to take my chances. Plus exercise and HRT will reduce my rate of colon cancer by 37 percent—an additional benefit."

The next time I asked how she was doing, she said she was still on her hormones. "And this time I will not be coming off! I had an epiphany, and I said to my husband, if I told you that by cutting off your testosterone production you would never have to fear the risk of prostate or testicular cancer, would you do it?" She explained to him that would be equivalent to her estrogen-deficiency state. He hasn't bothered her since. "Now he gets it," she said with a smile.

This demonstrates the value of conquering fear through research and knowledge. It also highlights the power of prevailing societal notions and the challenge of making decisions and taking responsibility for one's own health and wellness. If a medical doctor in the field of women's health, with her access to all the medical journals and information, still has such a difficult time with deciding about hormones, what is the average woman supposed to do?

Where does she seek information and, ultimately, guidance? I believe *Lifting the Veil* will help.

Are Hormones Safe?

Is coffee good for you? Then why do you drink it? Did you know people have died from caffeine overdose and that it can cause gastritis, which can lead to bleeding in the stomach? It can also cause a rapid heart rate and worsen hypertension.

If I guaranteed you that by staying home you would *never* have a car accident, would you give up driving? Of course not. When you get in your car every morning you don't agonize over the idea of a reckless driver coming around the corner. You drive your car and don't give it a second thought because you have places to go and things to do. Did you know your chances of coming to harm in the car are far greater than the risk of taking hormones?

So will you drive or play it safe and never go outside? You will never have an accident, but you are also guaranteed not to have a life.

When you drive your car you take prudent measures to obey the rules of the road, you service your car, and you are proactive. The more proactive you are about taking care of your car the more comfortable you are. This applies to everything. The better the information you have, the better prepared you are. This does not eliminate risk, but you are reassured that you did your due diligence.

If you watch the news on TV, it is packed with violence and death because that is what sells. If every show had a happy-ever-after story with no drama, no one would watch. Bad news sells commercials and rivets your attention. Don't you sometimes feel duped, manipulated, and maybe even addicted to the news? And to fear?

There is so much stuff advertised on TV it's hard to know what is right for you—what you *really* need. Intimidated with misinformation and "facts," it is no wonder you're afraid and uncertain as to what you can do for your symptoms. Let's be clear: you are being manipulated on all sides.

What about cancer? you ask. This is a good question, and one I am asked all the time. Nothing scares more people away from taking hormones than the fear of cancer.

"Cancer, cancer, cancer!" Bad news travels fast, and negative spins magnetically attract our attention. Everyone has a horror story; we are drowning in cancer news. It taps loudly at our fear of death. Often the underlying message is, you may get cancer or it may not be found soon enough and then it may not be curable. Be afraid. Be *very* afraid!

I know this is one of the biggest fears women have when they hear the word hormone. What we can challenge this with is science (see chapter 7 regarding studies). Hormones do not cause cancer, even though hormone-responsive cancers like breast, uterine, and prostate cancers are thought to perhaps grow faster when given hormones. Cancer likes hormones as much as all the other cells in your body; it is like fertilizer. That is why you need to do your due diligence by having preventive measures like mammograms and pap smears.

The commercials never claim testosterone causes prostate cancer yet the relationship is the same. So men take *their* testosterone happily, without fear.

Here's how the science of statistics works in medicine. There are research studies that are done that take facts and experience into account to help us come up with answers. I have written a separate chapter on the results of some of the major studies related to HRT and menopause.

Under ordinary circumstances, medical researchers help us by looking at the numbers and publishing them. Their work often helps us (e.g., reports on the ill effects of cigarette smoking, pollution, pesticides, endocrine disruptors, etc.) to figure out the cause of poor health. In the case of hormones, perhaps they drew some conclusions that led us astray. That happens sometimes, particularly when the results are skewed or the interpretation of the study are erroneous.

One of the pivotal studies causing fear regarding hormones was the Women's Health Initiative (WHI), which is discussed in chapter 7. The original WHI study results fanned the flames of fear, but when after a few years the dust settled, and the scientific community came to different conclusions (which discounted many of the earlier conclusions about risks), the general public never got the message.

Let's talk about breast cancer, which is the main cancer women fear most in relation to hormones. This is understandable since it is rampant in the United States. In fact, one in nine women will get it if they live to eighty-five. This is an amazing statistic, and it's not static. When I finished medical school it was one in twelve; when I started practice a decade later it was one in ten, and now it is one in nine.

Breast cancer is inarguably a risk for all women, whether they are on hormones or not. But there is no hard evidence that bioidentical estrogen or progesterone is going to *significantly* increase that risk. In fact, some experts believe that by taking the form of estrogen known as *estriol* (E3), you are actually lowering your risk because it protects the breast by suppressing proliferation (multiplying) of the cells.

Think about this: most cases of breast cancer occur in women after their hormone levels begin to decline. If estrogen is so bad for you, wouldn't cancer rates peak when women had their highest levels of estrogen—in their twenties and thirties?

Fewer than 5 percent of the cases of breast cancer are genetic, which obviously means 95 percent are not. They are possibly environmental. Therefore, even if someone in your family had breast cancer, you can't know if it was hereditary or environmentally caused. If the latter, then it doesn't affect your personal risk.

The only way to know if you might be one of the 5 percent is to do genetic testing. There have been articles calling for all women to be routinely tested at age thirty for the BRCA genes (the genes whose mutations are associated with higher risk of breast and ovarian cancers), but so far this has not gained much traction. It would be expensive for the health-insurance companies.

Certainly ask your doctor for the test if you are worried. If there are certain suspicious cancers in your family, I would recommend doing genetic counseling and testing. The key to any cancer is if you can't prevent it, catch it early and take care of it. If you do have a hormone-responsive cancer, it is true that hormones may make it grow faster, but so can oral contraceptive pills and a host of other factors. This is why I insist that all my patients do regular health maintenance to pick up any disease in its earliest stage.

Every woman should have regular pap smears, breast exams, and mammograms. They can also do thermograms (an imaging test for the breast that does not involve radiation or touching the breasts) if they choose. Once you have done these tests, rather than live in fear of the unknown, focus on being healthy and feeling well.

Remember these two realities: your risk of developing a hormone-dependent cancer is lower than your risk of having a heart attack. Heart disease is the leading cause of death in women. There is no evidence BHRT causes either.

Fear of cancer can be rational or irrational. For example, a patient of mine who happens to be a registered nurse decided to have her ovaries (but not her breasts) removed because she had a close relative who had ovarian cancer. That could be considered a rational mode of action, but she chose *not* to get the blood test that would show whether she had the gene that put her at increased risk of ovarian cancer. Despite having no problems, she just "wanted them out." (Having the blood test could also provide useful information for her daughter).

This may seem irrational since it does not guarantee she will not die from anything else, and it wasn't a sure bet that she would later on have a problem with her ovaries since they were perfectly fine at the time they were removed.

At the same time it seemed rational to her because of her degree of fear and the fact that she would not feel safe until she removed them. This is what she needed to do for herself, and I respect that, although I did not recommend it.

What about People Who Have Already Had Cancer?

"Ella" is a fifty-two-year-old woman with a history of breast cancer. She works in the health-care field and had done a lot of reading on hormones and cancer research. She and her husband had not been able to have intercourse for years because her cancer treatment caused her to go into menopause, resulting in severe vaginal dryness. She had a lot of stress at home with teenage kids, work, and a need to keep up appearances. Despite being a cancer survivor she was the one being strong for everyone else. By making sure she didn't burden anyone else, she increased her burden. Despite having no more breast tissue as a result of a double mastectomy, no doctor would give her hormones just because she'd had breast cancer. She was miserable.

On her first follow-up visit after we started to correct her imbalances, I asked her how she was doing. "I have been numb for years, but for the first time I am able to cry—you know, the good cry."

To me her response was profound. Like a typical doctor I was expecting a more concrete answer or quantification of her symptoms.

Ella's goal was simple: "I want to be able to have sex with my husband on Valentine's Day. I have defeated death, and now I need to have a life," she said, smiling. She had absolutely no fear of taking hormones; her only challenge was to find them. She is on them now and doing very well.

Fear Not!

Most books waffle when it comes to the subject of hormone replacement. They may extol the benefits of hormone replacement, but they never come out and categorically say it's safe. Patients need to hear that simple fact from their doctors. Hormones prescribed by a trained practitioner are safe and, when used appropriately, are actually safer than most medications. They may not be appropriate for everyone, but for the vast majority of women they are.

Do not let fear keep you from improving the quality of your life.

Menopause Myths

- If you ignore it, it will go away.
- There is nothing you can do about it.
- Menopause symptoms only last a year.
- Only self-indulgent or weak women have symptoms.
- It's embarrassing!
- It signals the end of a woman's productive life.
- It's a gyn problem.
- Your doctor probably knows more than you about this issue.
- Bioidentical hormones cause cancer.
- Menopause is only a woman's issue.
- It can't be menopause if you are still having periods.
- Menopause only happens to "old" women.
- Birth-control pills are safer than bioidentical hormones.
- It's not normal to want sex after menopause.
- Sex is not pleasurable after menopause, so your best bet is to avoid it!
- You can bypass menopause by having a hysterectomy.
- Hormones just delay menopause, but you still have to go through it.
- Most women have no symptoms.
- Taking hormones will make you start your periods again.
- It's not "natural" to treat menopause.

From: Insurance company pharmacy ES
Date: September 4, 2014

Dear Colleague

You recently prescribed a compounded drug for at least one of your patients. It contains ingredients not covered by your patient's prescription plan, which means your patient may be paying the medication's full cost.

As you know, compounded drugs, unlike FDA-approved drugs, often lack the rigorous, well-designed clinical studies to validate the safety and effectiveness of consistent strengths, quantities and combinations. Also, the cost for some compound ingredients has risen by as much as 1000%.

With this in mind, please consider prescribing a commercially available, FDA-approved medication.

If you do prescribe a compounded drug and your patient chooses to appeal the decision to deny coverage, your patient will be asked to contact you in an effort to gain approval for coverage. You in turn, need to provide published medical data and documented evidence that similar *commercially available* medication has failed to or will not help this patient.

We appreciate your consideration and evaluation.

Sincerely,
A.R. B, Doctor of Pharmacy
ES

"ES manages the prescription benefit for your patients at the request of their employer, plan sponsor or health plan

****

NADU A. TUAKLI, MD, MPH

Chapter 2

The Role of Hormones
in Women

Look deep into nature, and then you will
understand everything better.
—Albert Einstein

WE COULD NOT survive without hormones. They are "chemical messengers" that perform their amazing tasks from head to toe 24/7. They help children grow and determine when puberty occurs and when we become adults. They have regulating roles including controlling body temperature, blood pressure, and blood sugar levels. They determine when a woman has a period and when she goes into menopause. They stimulate and manage all the functions of all the organs in the body.

Hormones are made by specialized organs called glands. Examples of glands are the pituitary, thyroid, adrenals, ovaries, and testes, and they all release hormones into the blood when needed.

Given the fact that hormones control every process that goes on inside you, have you paid enough attention to them over the years? We cannot survive without hormones. They are vital chemical messengers. Ideally we should all have had our baseline hormone levels checked before age thirty-five because that is when they gradually start to decline. Almost all of the hormones in the body decrease with aging.

Cortisol is generally an exception to the rule and often increases. Cortisol is a steroid hormone that is formed from the same pathway as the sex hormones. It is often called the stress hormone because it is responsible for your fight-or-flight response in a stressful situation.

Most modern-day women churn out way too much cortisol. This has its own downside because the adrenals are working so hard it can lead to a condition called adrenal fatigue. It is considered adrenal burnout when the adrenals just can't make any more cortisol.

There are other hormones that come from the same pathway, like aldosterone, which controls your salt and water balance and related things like blood pressure.

Hormones like estrogen, progesterone, growth hormone, melatonin, testosterone DHEA, and so on all decline after age thirty-five. What can make a big difference to your well-being is the *rate* at which the hormones decrease. If they drop too rapidly you may not have as easy a transition as someone who has a gradual rate of decline. This is what happens, for example, when the ovaries are removed with a hysterectomy. The hormone levels plummet.

Most situations are not that drastic, but the bottom line is that universally every fifty-year-old has a lower hormone level than they did at thirty-five. When the hormones get to a suboptimal level, symptoms begin (see chapter 4 for the symptoms).

The slope of hormone decline after 35 can determine the severity of symptoms

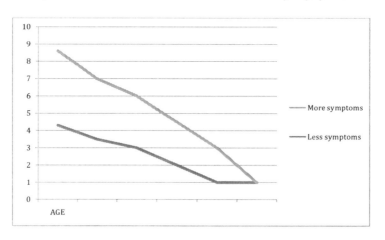

Hormone Decline over age

NADU A. TUAKLI, MD, MPH

How Do These "Messenger Hormones" Work?

Once a gland produces a hormone, it travels to distant organs to find its own specific receptors. Think of a lock and key system. The receptor (lock) stays in the locked position until the hormone (key) arrives. When a hormone comes upon a specific "lock," it unlocks it and activates the cell's function. For example, if the cell's function is to make you sneeze, you will sneeze!

LOCK AND KEY MECHANISM

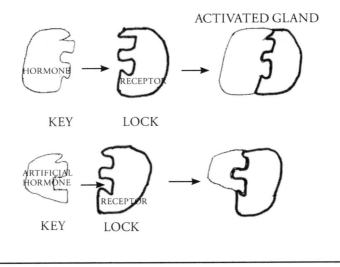

ACTIVATED GLAND

KEY   LOCK

KEY   LOCK

Artificial Hormones create jigsaw pieces that don't quite fit

---

Sometimes the cell's function is to release another hormone of its own. This is how the thyroid works when it gets messages from the brain. *All* hormones work in this fashion.

To prevent overproduction of hormones, there is a feedback mechanism that tells the brain there is enough circulating hormone, and then the brain sends out a different hormone to shut it off.

Synthetic hormones, as with many drugs, can also activate organs by acting as fake keys. Many medications, such as some for blood pressure, are designed to work by blocking various receptors. On the other hand, the *inadvertent* blocking of receptors is also what causes the side effects of a lot of medications. Some cancer drugs work by locking receptors on the out-of-control cells so they cannot multiply. Thus, balancing both the positive and negative (proactive and reactive) receptors of cells is critical. The ultimate controller is always the brain.

There is a receptor for both estrogen and progesterone on *every* cell in the body. All hormones interact with and depend on each other. There are two main types of hormones in the body: steroidal and nonsteroidal.

The steroid group is formed from cholesterol. The other group of hormones are not cholesterol-related. Examples of nonsteroidal hormones are insulin, thyroid, and growth hormone.

For the purposes of this book, I concentrate on the steroidal hormones that govern menopause. These include estrogen, testosterone, progesterone, and DHEA. (See the "Steroidal Hormone" chart below showing that they are all derived from cholesterol via pregnenolone.)

STEROID PATHWAY

Hormones made from cholesterol

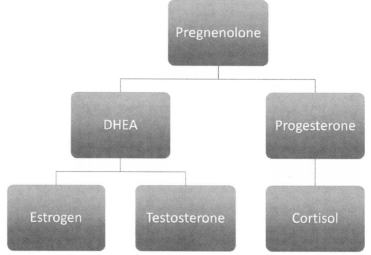

If your cholesterol is too low you can't make estrogen *or* testosterone. It is important to understand that menopause causes many different hormonal derangements. In addition it tends to occur around the time that other glands, like the thyroid and adrenal, may be decreasing their output as well. All these combined can make one feel "out of whack."

In the reproductive years, the ovaries produce most of the estrogen, progesterone, and testosterone in the body. When they stop producing eggs, hormone production is whittled down to miniscule levels.

As noted in chapter 3, the perimenopausal phase is a tumultuous time. Almost all the symptoms of menopause are due to this decreased production and relative deficiency. When the brain detects that the ovaries are not making as much hormone as they used to, it starts to increase messenger hormones in an attempt to get the ovaries to work harder. The messenger hormones are luteinizing hormone (LH) and follicle-stimulating hormone (FSH). An elevated level of either tends to indicate that the corresponding organ is not working adequately. This is why these two hormones are often used as a diagnostic test to see if a woman is menopausal. It is reliable in postmenopausal women but not in perimenopause because the levels are fluctuating wildly.

Interestingly enough, men have these two hormones as well, but in men their job is to make the testicles work properly. Men who have sexual dysfunction should also have these hormones checked.

The fact that there is an estrogen and progesterone receptor in every cell in the body gives you an idea of how widespread the action of these hormones is and why the syndrome of menopause affects so many different organ systems.

The ratio between estrogen and progesterone is very important and needs to be maintained. Consider them the yin and yang. Science hasn't yet figured out why some of those organs, such as the tongue or eyeball, need receptors for them, but I'm sure we will eventually find out.

Testosterone similarly has a lot of different actions in the muscles, the brain, and the bones as well as in the blood.

Estrogen: the Yin

TYPES OF HUMAN ESTROGEN
ESTRONE E1
ESTRADIOL E2
ESTRIOL   E3

Human estrogen is actually many different estrogen hormones the three main estrogens are estrone (E1), estradiol (E2), and estriol (E3). For overall balance and optimum well–being, estrogen must always be balanced by progesterone. It makes absolutely no sense to give a woman only estrogen as a hormone replacement for menopause, because just adding estrogen will throw the body further off balance.

Many of my gyn colleagues feel that if a woman doesn't have a uterus, she does not need progesterone. Their argument is that if she has no uterus she can't get uterine cancer. Well we figured that out without a medical degree. The problem as I see it is that there is more to a woman than a uterus.

What about the brain and the nervous system and all the other organs in the body that have estrogen and progesterone receptors? Most perimenopausal and menopausal women are not making sufficient amounts of progesterone. When you give a woman who is already estrogen dominant unopposed estrogen, you make her situation worse. The breasts are bombarded with estrogen with no "yang" to balance it. This can lead to sore breasts and encourage random cancerous cells in the breasts as well as in the uterus to multiply.

Women with estrogen dominance may have "exaggerated" menopause, if you will, and may have episodes of irregular bleeding. You can have estrogen dominance because of an unbalanced ratio of estrogen to progesterone even if overall the total amount of estrogen is deficient. You can be both estrogen dominant and deficient at the same time.

I don't agree with the prevailing Western medical "wisdom" that views the risk of uterine cancer as the sole means of determining whether a woman "deserves" progesterone.

Hopefully one day medical science will catch up with nature and emulate its wonderful ability to create balance. More on this in greater detail when we discuss bioidentical hormone-replacement therapy.

Important functions of estrogen include

- regulating ovulation and periods
- stimulating bone-building cells
- normal brain function
- vaginal lubrication
- mood stability
- maintaining moisture of membranes, including skin

Estrogens are generally derived from testosterone and androstenedione in the ovaries by a process called aromatization.

The three estrogens (E1, E2, E3; see above) are slightly different in their functioning.

E1 is estrone, which is considered more stimulatory to the breasts than the others meaning it can cause proliferation of breast tissue. This is the predominant estrogen in menopause and can be converted from estradiol and vice versa. Fat cells produce estrogen, mostly E1, so extra weight can lead to excess estrogen and estrogen dominance.

Prior to menopause, 80 percent of estrogen is estradiol, or E2. After menopause it drops down to a very low but constant level. E2 is made in the ovaries and is the most potent of the naturally occurring estrogens.

Estriol is E3. It is not made in the ovaries but is generated in the placenta or from the conversion of E2 and E1. It is the weakest of all the estrogens and does not stimulate the breasts. It is thought to offer protection against breast cancer. Large amounts of this are made during pregnancy and are known to protect against multiple sclerosis flare-ups.

Now we come to estrogen-like products: Premarin is made from the urine of pregnant horses and is often referred to as an estrogen, which is partly true. The problem is that it is *equine* estrogen. Neigh! It bears no resemblance to any of the three human (bioidentical) estrogens except that it can act as a fake key and unlock human estrogen receptors throughout the body.

Because everything that enters the body is broken down by the liver, foreign substances also create odd breakdown products never seen before in addition to the initial foreign substance. This is how abnormal substances result in the system going haywire.

If you're lucky your system can tolerate horse estrogen and will obey the commands (keys) just as if it were human estrogen. However, if you are unlucky, the introduction of unrecognized estrogens can make you feel unwell. The famous study called the Women's Health Initiative Study (in 2002) showed evidence of this. It was a study of thousands of women on "estrogen" and because it was sponsored by Wyeth, which was the pharmaceutical company that made Premarin, Prempro, and Provera, only their products (i.e., equine estrogen and medroxyprogesterone) were used. They succeeded in proving that synthetic hormones are bad for women (see chapter 7), but unfortunately this also left women with the idea that all hormones are bad.

There is a wide range of other hormone imbalances that cause a lot of symptoms, so feeling bad is not always due to estrogen deficiency. Progesterone, thyroid, and adrenal gland hormones (like cortisol) can also be out of balance, resulting in a lot of distress and discomfort. There are also the two building blocks, DHEA and pregnenolone, which may need to be supplemented. (See the chart on steroidal hormone synthesis on page 16.)

Progesterone: the Yang

Only one progesterone is made by humans, and that is simple progesterone. Unfortunately there are several "progestins" made by pharmaceutical companies. These chemicals act like keys on the progesterone receptors and are named to sound like progesterone. This can confuse the user, but no matter how similar the name, remember this: it's only real progesterone if it's called *progesterone*. If you look at a label and it says Progestin, medroxyprogesterone, Provera, or any other "pro," it is not *progesterone,* and it has little or no resemblance to real progesterone. The names are actually more similar than the chemical structures.

Chemicals in this group include medroxyprogesterone, otherwise known as Provera, Progestasert, or a host of other ones used in birth-control pills. Examples of progestins can be seen below:

EVERYDAY PROGESTINS
Levonorgestrel (Mirena, Plan B, Norplant, Contraceptive pills)
Medroxyprogesterone (Provera, Depo Provera)
Norethindrone (Contraceptive pills)
Norgestimate (Contraceptive pills)

As mentioned earlier, when the body breaks down foreign substances like these, it's not just the initial foreign substance that can cause problems. The body doesn't recognize the metabolites either.

Besides balancing estrogen, important functions of natural progesterone include

FUNCTIONS OF PROGESTERONE
Balances estrogen
Enhances and stabilizes mood
Calms
Supports other endocrine glands
Rebuilds bone
Protects the uterine lining
Promotes restful sleep

Progesterone is not just needed by postmenopausal women. In fact, it is one of the major players in premenstrual syndrome (PMS). Most women who suffer from PMS have a progesterone deficiency. It is the lack of progesterone that causes the irritability, bloating, menstrual disturbances, and depression along with the other symptoms.

In my view, giving a woman progesterone just to prevent her from getting uterine cancer is an extremely narrow and myopic view of managing a woman's health. The purpose of giving a woman progesterone is to correct her body's deficiency and thereby improve her overall health and quality of life.

Testosterone

Testosterone is another hormone that is significantly lacking after menopause. It is good for you because it can increase estrogen, boost libido, prevent osteoporosis, increase bone and muscle strength, and improve memory and mental acuity. The most famous hormone for improving libido is testosterone, but it is by no means the only player. Estrogen, DHEA, and progesterone all have a role to play.

Testosterone is made by the ovaries and the adrenal gland and by conversion from other hormones. The ovaries continue to make testosterone after menopause but in much smaller amounts, and low levels of this hormone are associated with decreased libido. As will be discussed in chapter 5, many factors affect the libido, so for maximum relief *you need to address them all*. What's interesting is that there really isn't a normal blood range of testosterone for postmenopausal women. This is because it varies so much and because people's level of arousal does not directly correlate with the levels of this hormone in their blood. Furthermore, testosterone is not effective if a woman is lacking estrogen and progesterone.

As an aside: Men also suffer from hormone deficiency. "Andropause" is often referred to as male menopause. This is a state in which a man's hormones are imbalanced, and he may suffer decreased libido, decreased sexual function, fatigue, loss of muscle mass, and depression. Some men describe it as a feeling of "sudden" aging. Once again this is usually multifaceted, but is predominantly associated with a lack of testosterone.

One of the easiest and most accurate ways to measure your hormone levels and to determine what needs to be adjusted is saliva testing. A saliva test is done with a kit furnished by your doctor. Four samples are taken throughout the day to account for the hormone fluctuation during daily activities. An advantage of the saliva test over a blood test is that it reflects what the levels of the hormones are at the tissue level, and it takes into account the diurnal (day cycle) changes. It is the most accurate test for determining perimenopause.

The New Normal

Have you ever been told that your results are "normal," yet you feel awful? Maybe what is considered normal is actually not normal for you. "Normal ranges" have varied a lot with time. For example, blood sugar and blood pressure guidelines have varied greatly over the years.

A normal fasting blood sugar has gradually decreased from 125 to 99. Twenty years ago a blood pressure of 140/90 was considered normal, and now that is classified as mild hypertension and an optimal BP is 120/80.

The real question is how to determine your own normal, and this is one of the reasons it is good to get baseline measures before age thirty-five.

SUMMARY

Hormones take messages from one part of the body to another. Now that you understand who the players are, let's recap.

There are different kinds of hormones, and they have important jobs. One of these jobs is to make you feel good and function well. Menopause occurs because the ovaries "retire" and stop making some hormones.

Perimenopause is the semiretirement phase during which women may have low libido, fatigue, anxiety, depression, and weight gain. They may also experience autoimmune symptoms, thyroid dysfunction, joint pain, and allergies.

Menopause is essentially a deficiency state; lack of these hormones affects every single organ in the body.

You have the option to do nothing or you can choose to replace what you have lost. You can replace them with biochemically similar hormones and try to emulate nature, or you can replace them with synthetic "keys."

I believe bioidentical hormone replacement is not rocket science. For people who have uncomfortable symptoms from menopause, the idea is to replace hormones that are identical to what the ovaries used to make, thus eliminating the symptoms while improving the quality of life of the individual.

Types of Human Estrogen

- **Estrone (E1)**
- **Estradiol (E2)**
- **Estriol (E3)**

Functions of Estrogen

- prepares the uterus for pregnancy
- regulates menstruation
- maintains mood and memory
- maintains moisture
- protects against osteoporosis

Functions of Progesterone

- balances estrogen
- enhances and stabilizes mood
- calming
- supports other endocrine systems
- rebuilds bone
- protects uterine lining
- restful sleep

> You can be both estrogen deficient and estrogen dominant at the same time

> Most PMS sufferers have a deficiency of progesterone

Chapter 3

Meet the "Pauses": Menopause, Perimenopause, and Postmenopause

The only thing that is constant is change.
—Heraclitus, a Greek Philosopher

The Veil

WHY DOES MENOPAUSE carry such a massive social stigma? A stigma so significant it creates a huge barrier that stops many from getting the help they need. The stigma is persistent; it taps into what many consider a taboo to discuss, and other social conventions.

This taboo has not evolved much in the twenty-first century the way other topics have. For example, we now speak more freely about sex, gender, and mental-health issues. But still there remains an unspoken request not to discuss things to do with menstrual periods and hormonal changes in women.

Mothers rarely share their experiences of menopause with their daughters. Women are hesitant to admit to their girlfriends that they are menopausal.

A patient once explained to me why she and her girlfriends don't discuss the subject. "Menopause is not 'diva-ish'," she says.

The shroud of menopause envelopes doctors and medical education in general, so students, patients, partners, and their families are all part of this big taboo. We don't teach about it, and we barely acknowledge its existence. The prevailing wisdom is that it would be so much more convenient if it would just go away and quickly.

The problem has been exacerbated by the scientific and medical community that refuses to acknowledge that menopause is a *valid* condition that can be debilitating for some women. Too many doctors view menopause as a "quasi-condition," implying it is just a natural process that women go through and not really worthy of a lot of time or discussion. They did not receive information about it in medical school and have no desire to learn about it now. As a result, they continue to perpetuate the conventional way of handling it, which is to either ignore it or provide "shotgun medication" and wait it out.

These doctors who have pledged to "do no harm" often make women's situations worse by offering them antidepressants or tranquilizers or telling them they're just too young to have hormonal problems. Yet they have no qualms about giving synthetic hormones that cause additional side effects or redirecting the patient to a psychiatrist.

Courtroom Drama

Mandy had been a highly successful attorney with her own practice for years, but by the time she came to see me, her legal career was almost in ruins, thanks to the brain fog, anxiety, and insomnia inflicted by perimenopause. She was a highly educated woman, but in spite of this she was misdiagnosed and overmedicated and was at her wits' end. As I later discovered, the solution to her problem was a simple remedy that completely cleared up her symptoms. Yet the ordeal she'd suffered before finally getting relief almost ran her, her family, and her business off the rails. Since then, things have not gotten much better for women like Mandy.

Here is a dramatization of her story.

The *overweight* woman was a little breathless as she slowly made her way up to the front of the hushed courtroom. As a result of the bailiff's command, it was quiet enough to hear the swishing sound her pantyhose made with each step as her heavy thighs rubbed against each other. The effort of walking to the front of the court had left her a little *breathless,* and she could feel *palpitations* starting. These symptoms were nothing new; they were her "new normal."

Mandy, forty-one, was there to represent her client. As usual, getting ready for court that morning wasn't easy. Despite her medications, new symptoms and fresh obstacles seemed to arise daily, and those, coupled with a three-year-old son, made her *exhausted* before the day started. It just seemed to be getting harder and harder to keep the pieces of her life together.

She had gotten married a few years before. Some might consider her a late starter, but at least she had acquired her professional credentials, of which she was justly proud. And here she was center stage, a private-practice lawyer doing her "thing."

Her usual dramatic courtroom flare had taken a hit over the past several months, but at least she was still functional, she thought. Besides, she figured at some point she would get used to her habitual *tiredness.* But what the heck? She looked to the side and her client looked back eagerly, anxious to get started. She looked up at the bench, indicating to the judge that she was ready.

The judge returned her gaze and said, "Okay, Counselor, state your case."

There was nothing unfamiliar about this request, yet all of a sudden her *mind was blank.* Words danced on the page in front of her, but she could not remember anything. Mortified, Mandy struggled to remember the details of the case she was here to present.

"I can't live like this," Mandy blurted out to me a few days later as she narrated in great detail the humiliating events of that court episode. She wanted me to help her understand how she had arrived at such a low point. "They keep telling me I am too young to be menopausal, but I know I'm not crazy. It has to be hormonal."

She told me she had been feeling "different" for quite some time. She couldn't predict what specific symptoms she would have on any given day, but she noted *lack of sleep, fatigue,* and *irregular periods* over the past year. She was having a hard time sleeping and felt *anxious* at times.

She had gone to her gynecologist (gyn) several times with these complaints and had asked the doctor if she thought perhaps Mandy was menopausal. Her gyn told her that the few tests she had reluctantly run confirmed she was not menopausal.

After a couple more visits, the gyn recommended that perhaps Mandy would feel better if she took something for sleep and gave her a prescription for a sleep medication. The doctor recommended Mandy work on her stress levels. This did not help, and Mandy started to become anxious, knowing something was very wrong.

"You should see a psychiatrist," her gyn recommended.

Mandy followed instructions. She saw the psychiatrist and was given a tranquilizer and referred for psychotherapy.

When things did not improve the patient started to feel so *depressed* about her condition that her mental-health professionals felt she should also take an antidepressant. The triple combo of medications for sleep, anxiety, and depression resulted in a *surreal* feeling in addition to worsening her fatigue.

Despite being groggy, *fuzzy,* and depressed, Mandy tried to function as a mother and still went to work—until now. "I can't live like this! I can't function. I'm miserable."

(The italicized symptoms above are all clues of hormonal imbalance issues, which will be explained in the following chapters.)

I reassured the patient that even though a little premature, there were many women who started perimenopause at forty-one. I validated her concerns and her feelings and said it certainly could be physical. She was just relieved to have someone listen to her, and she was right about her symptoms being related to a hormone imbalance. As it turned out, she definitely was perimenopausal. Her progesterone level was undetectable in her blood test, and once I gave her the appropriate progesterone cream she was able to stop all the medications and resume her normal professional life. She is still in private practice today.

This was actually a pivotal case for me because here was an educated woman who was misdiagnosed and whose life was near crisis point by the time she realized she could talk to me, her primary-care physician (PCP). She had already seen two other doctors and was on various medications by the time she came to me as her seemingly last resort.

Besides reflecting a general misunderstanding of the skills family practitioners offer, it also made me become interested in the hormonal issues of women and how they are underdiagnosed and mistreated. If an educated woman like Mandy did not have access to this information, what about those with fewer resources?

This scenario could have ended very differently. This was a successful professional woman being put out to pasture for "mental-health problems" while her life as she knew it was ending, a move enabled by the medical community that was supposed to help her.

How could this happen?

One of the reasons is the lack of knowledge both in the lay community as well as the medical community about menopause. The fact is that in many medical schools not even a single lecture is dedicated to menopause. It is considered a quasi-condition, "just" a natural process that women go through and not really worthy of a lot of time or discussion.

I believe that in many ways, the symptoms of perimenopause are much harder on women than the symptoms of menopause. This is because it is harder to diagnose; oftentimes the woman is still having periods, and she gets brushed off as if the problem is all psychological. Sometimes women are glad to see the onset of hot flashes and lack of periods just to be able to prove that they actually have a problem. I'm convinced that many instances of "midlife crisis" are actually cases of perimenopause.

Four Stages

There are four stages in a woman's natural lifecycle. They are loosely defined by the activity of her menstrual cycle.

1. **Premenopause** is the period after menstruation begins at puberty. (The actual onset of having periods is called menarche.)
2. **Perimenopause** is the transition from the reproductive state into menopause. This is when ovulation is winding down but the woman is still menstruating. It is similar to menopause in

the sense that it is a time of hormone imbalance, and a lot of what is true about menopause is also true for perimenopause.

3. **Menopause** is the time during which periods cease completely and there is no further ovulation.

4. **Postmenopause** is the time after which there has been no period for a year.

Many women think that if they can get through the twelve months after menopause, all their symptoms will magically disappear. This is a myth. Symptoms may get progressively worse, and oftentimes it's around the one-year mark that women come to realize they need to take action.

Some women can ignore perimenopause and menopause and get by without taking any remedies for it, but others aren't so lucky.

Perimenopause

Perimenopause is the transitional period leading up to menopause and can occur ten years or more before menopause actually happens. Perimenopause is a time when progesterone production particularly becomes erratic before shutting down completely.

The lack of support during this time, particularly from physicians, is a major source of stress for many patients. Many people don't know perimenopause can actually be a rougher time for women than menopause itself. Reasons for this include the following:

1. The woman is still having periods so everyone, including doctors, tend to assume her hormonal system is still functioning the same way it used to. Often the perimenopausal woman may be mystified as to why she feels so lousy because she doesn't realize her symptoms are hormone-related.

2. The body is just beginning to get used to the varying levels of hormones after having had constant amounts for almost forty years, and it is essentially rebelling. In addition to overall lower levels, it is also adjusting to changing levels throughout the day. There are fluctuations on a day-to-day basis. No two days are

the same, and the hormones can even fluctuate hourly. The ups and downs are particularly trying, both emotionally and energy-wise.

3. With the daily fluctuations in hormone levels, a woman doesn't know when she wakes up in the morning what kind of day it's going to be. It could be anywhere between a deficiency day or a day on hormone overdrive.

4. To make things worse, the classic blood tests for menopause may not show any changes at all (unless you time the blood draw perfectly), so the symptoms are often assumed to be more psychological than physical.

5. Then there is the lack of diagnostic criteria. Most women did not check their baseline levels of hormones at thirty-five, so later, when they are symptomatic, they check these hormones and they appear to be within "normal" limits. The problem is, what is normal? Normal for you may not be the same as the population at large. If you do not know what your levels were when you were younger, there really is no way to determine how much they have changed.

In the next chapter you will understand just how powerful hormones are and why all these changes can make you feel physically ill.

In my experience perimenopause is the time when patients are most commonly misdiagnosed. The patient complaining about insomnia is given a sleeping pill, but she returns worried because she's feeling a lot worse, but then she gets some pills for anxiety. Her primary care physician (PCP) may refer her to a psychiatrist and perhaps for the first time in her life she is diagnosed with mental-health issues like depression. This occurs similarly with other "unexplained" symptoms.

It never ceases to amaze me how many people readily take Prozac and birth-control pills (which are equivalent to relatively large hormone doses) yet turn green at the thought of taking a bioidentical hormone for menopause. You can certainly take as many pills for your condition as you wish, but be aware that it is not more "natural" to take prescription psychotropic pharmaceuticals instead of bioidentical hormones, which are chemically identical to what your body makes itself.

Perimenopause is the time when menstrual irregularities are most prominent. So it is a peak time to perform hysterectomies (the median age is 40.9, per the Centers for Disease Control and Prevention). As a result of the roller-coaster hormones, a woman may skip menstrual cycles or, on the other hand, she may bleed incessantly. The woman and the doctor finally give up and remove the uterus because of prolonged bleeding. Fibroids, which are very common (more than 70 percent of women older than fifty have them), are often assumed to be the cause of the bleeding, so they end up as the official reason for the hysterectomy. Just under half a million hysterectomies (down from six hundred thousand) are performed annually in the United States, 86 percent for benign reasons. Of course a hysterectomy often involves removal of the fallopian tubes as well, but hopefully not the ovaries.

Removal of the ovaries increases a woman's risk of death from all causes by 8.6 percent if they are removed by age fifty-five and 3.9 percent if they are removed by fifty-nine. The numbers increase if they are removed at an even younger age. [68, 69]

The uterus and fallopian tubes are not just static tube structures that act as conduits for eggs; they secrete various hormones and secretions themselves. This is why many women notice changes after surgery (e.g., tubal ligations) even if their ovaries are left in place. In some women, pelvic surgery causes them to become menopausal sooner.

On the other hand, surgery may not be necessary, and the bleeding in many cases can be controlled with hormonal manipulation. This is why gynecologists often put patients on birth-control pills or insert an IUD laced with progestins hoping to control it. One of the problems with these types of hormones is that they are totally synthetic and can increase your risk of breast cancer, hypertension, and heart disease. The risk is even higher in smokers.

Menopause

The term menopause comes from a Greek word meaning the stopping of menstruation, even though the syndrome of menopause generally starts before that actually happens (perimenopause). The average

age of menopause is fifty-one but may occur as early as thirty-eight. Menopause prior to forty-five is considered premature.

Officially a woman is not considered menopausal until she has not had a period for one year. As with many things in medicine, this is just a definition, not a hard and fast rule. In some instances it is helpful, in others it is not. For example, a woman becomes menopausal immediately after having her ovaries removed no matter how young she is, so this definition would not apply in this case. Also, many women have symptoms long before that last period. In practical terms this definition is most useful in advising women that if it hasn't been a full year since their last period, they should not yet count their chickens. There is no guarantee they won't get another one.

The very word menopause can strike fear in women, even in those too young to really know what it is. It is a syndrome that continues to be misunderstood. Women intuitively know its impact can be dramatic, that it can change their self-concept as a woman, that it can destabilize a woman's quality of life and at its worst cripple a woman's ability to function. As an offshoot, this destabilization can also adversely impact her relationships with partners, friends, and family and even society as a whole.

Still, there are some definite positives to menopause, and not everyone is symptomatic. No woman can avoid going though menopause if she lives long enough, and there is no way to determine whether it is going to be easy or hard or even when it will occur.

You may get a clue from your mother's age at menopause, but this is variable. If you started menarche late you may have a later menopause, but this is not a hard and fast rule. As mentioned above, surgeries like tubal ligation may bring menopause on sooner.

So What Precisely Is Going on in the Body that Is Causing the Symptoms?

With each menstrual cycle the ovaries produce three main hormones: estrogen, testosterone, and progesterone, as well as an egg (ovulation). At the time of menopause the ovaries stop producing significant amounts of these hormones. In short, they pack up shop. This is a gradual process that doesn't happen overnight. Little by little the "inventory" decreases, and some months before the grand closing the ovaries may decide not to ovulate at all or just sporadically.

Once again think of progesterone and estrogen as the yin and the yang of your sexual organs (which includes your brain, by the way!). The balance between progesterone and estrogen is crucial to a feeling of well-being. As noted in chapter 2 there is a receptor for estrogen and progesterone in every cell in the body, even your eyes. Therefore, it is hardly surprising that menopause as a syndrome affects the entire body and all its systems (more on this in chapter 4). This is also the reason why simply taking care of one symptom such as vaginal lubrication may not result in feeling holistically optimal.

Despite popular conceptions to the contrary, menopause is a syndrome, not a symptom. How do these differ? A symptom is a single physical manifestation, a complaint that is observed without taking the cause into consideration. A syndrome, on the other hand, is a group of symptoms that all stem from a common cause. For example, a cough is a symptom, but when it is associated with a fever, body aches, nausea, vomiting, sore throat, runny nose, earache, etc., it becomes part of the syndrome of a cold or the flu. On the other hand, the same symptom (the cough) could also be part of other syndromes like allergies or lung cancer.

Similarly, menopause is not just about the symptom of hot flashes. The hormonal disruption it causes results in symptoms throughout a woman's body, creating the syndrome of menopause. The syndrome varies from person to person in terms of what symptoms each person has and also how the individual experiences it. In a nutshell, menopause is a deficiency syndrome—basically stuff you used to have you don't anymore. The body is acutely aware that it is now deficient in something and craves what it used to have.

Once the body grows accustomed to the absence of hormones, it will compensate and the symptoms will go away. If you're lucky, it will make the appropriate adjustments (tolerance) without too much discomfort.

Unfortunately, there is no general time frame for when this might happen. While some women adjust after a short period, perhaps a couple of years, some women may take twenty years or more. Everyone has symptoms, but just as with pain, individual tolerance varies. Some women have such mild symptoms they adjust very quickly, at least physically. On the other hand, there are some unfortunate women who just have a system that doesn't tolerate hormonal changes very well: they get postpartum depression, have severe PMS, experience traumatic perimenopause, and don't do well after menopause.

Sometimes the emotional changes are more significant than the physical ones. In some cultures the cessation of menstruation means a woman is essentially "dried up" and deemed less valuable than younger women. She may even be felt to be of no further use to society. The psychological impact is especially difficult if a woman's sense of self-worth is tied up with her ability to have children.

Does going through the change necessarily have to put you through changes? No. You can minimize any changes by knowing exactly what is going on and what your options are. Education is key.

Menopause does not need to be thought of as all gloom and doom. Far from it. Many women endure menopause, and once they are on the "other side," they say their lives are better and more fulfilled, especially if they have suffered from severe menstrual-related symptoms or had a lot of children to take care of.

The other positive aspects of this transition may include shrinkage of fibroids and the end of PMS and menstrual migraines.

Myth-Busters

Myth:
Menopause lasts a year and then it's over.

Fact:
Menopausal symptoms can go on for years and vary greatly from woman to woman.

Myth:
Menopause doesn't occur before age fifty.

Fact:
The date of menopause varies more widely than the age of menarche.
It can begin as early as the late thirties or as late as the late fifties.

Chapter 4

Symptoms of Hormonal Imbalance

Health is not merely the absence of disease
—WHO

HERE WE DISCUSS symptoms that can be experienced in menopause and how women may feel. I cannot tell you how many women have said to me, "I didn't realize how bad I felt until I felt better," or "I can't believe I waited so long to do something." One important reason people do nothing is that they lack information. They also get tired of being blown off by their doctors. One patient told me, "They made me feel ridiculous for even suggesting I might have a hormone imbalance."

There is a wide array of symptoms that results when hormones fluctuate, whether due to PMS, perimenopause, or menopause, or even a disorder like endometriosis. Not all women experience the same symptoms, if any at all, and certainly not to the same degree. Each person's experience is unique.

When you consider these symptoms against the backdrop of the demands of modern-day life, you can begin to see why, if not addressed properly, menopause can bring about a less-than-optimal state of well-being.

Many women in their forties and fifties multitask; they raise children, take care of aging parents, and still continue their careers. They start their day with an impressive to-do list. There are continual demands in all directions, and hectic schedules make it difficult to find time for reflection or for them to care for themselves. At the same time, our lifestyles create factors that place additional stress on our bodies. These include inadequate nutrients in our food, too many unhealthy calories, lack of physical activity, and toxins in the environment. All these factors disrupt hormonal balance, and then menopause is added on.

One hundred years ago, when a woman's life expectancy was forty seven, women didn't live long enough to worry about estrogen deficiency, but since then, life expectancy has nearly doubled and quality-of-life expectations have totally changed. On the other hand, our hormonal system has not adapted to a longer life span, so we still go through menopause at the same age.

In chapter 2, I discussed exactly what hormones are and why they are so important, but suffice it to say we humans are all about hormones: every process that goes on inside us is controlled by our hormones. Although it tends to be more apparent in women, there comes a point in the lives of *all* individuals when their hormonal levels change. Menopause is a time of hormone deficiency that affects the entire body.

Menopause can have a profound physical, emotional, and psychological impact on how we feel about ourselves and our partners. That every woman's symptoms are due to a change in hormone levels is a fact and a commonality. But how each woman responds to these changing levels varies greatly.

The same is true of pregnancy, a condition that is also governed by hormones: some women can tell immediately when they are pregnant, and others feel completely unchanged. Some have miserable morning sickness and others sail through, oblivious of discomfort. This is because some women are more affected by hormonal shifts than others, which is why menstrual patterns are so diverse.

So one of the basic things to understand about menopause is that it is fundamentally different for every woman, so it is impossible to describe every woman's symptoms. From woman to woman the biological physiology doesn't vary much, but the degree of hormonal fluctuation and the individual's response alters the experience. Because of the variation between women and even the change within the same person from month to month, treatment needs to be highly individualized.

The good news is that what you think you feel you can really own. It's not in your head; it is your specific menopause. Unfortunately, millions of women don't realize their myriad of symptoms are hormone-related, so they suffer in silence.

Is it in My Head? Can it Be My Hormones?

You don't have to have hot flashes to be menopausal.

Patients often ask worriedly if I think they might be menopausal because they haven't had a period. Because of all the horror stories, they continue on "high alert" for several years, waiting for something bad to happen. These are the lucky ones. On the other end of the spectrum are women who may have symptoms like hot flashes and insomnia that goes on for ten years or more. A lot depends on how a particular woman's body rebalances to the lack of hormones.

Women's perception of the severity of their symptoms also varies. Some have symptoms but still find them manageable, whereas some find the same symptoms intolerable. These are important considerations when determining a treatment path and deciding whether something actually needs to be done about the symptoms.

There is a common misconception that menopause is a gynecological problem when in fact most of the symptoms have nothing to do with the pelvic organs. The only real gynecological symptom of menopause is vaginal dryness. The endocrine disruption that menopause creates results in diverse symptoms that affect the brain, body temperature, memory, the ability to sleep, emotions, dizziness, and even joint pain, to name a few.

What Symptoms Will I Have?

Anything and everything that can go wrong—may! It is unlikely that as you go through menopause the only change you'll notice is that your periods have stopped. When it finally happens, only 10 percent of women report no other symptoms.

On the other hand, surveys show that 20 percent of women have no difficulty (although it's unclear how many of those women are downplaying their experience because of societal expectations), another 10 percent have minor incapacitation, and the remaining 70 percent have clear manifestations of hormone deficiency. That 70 percent represents millions of women.

As a physician it is part of my job to validate how a patient feels. I never say, "Oh no, that's not possible; you're too young for that," or "It can't be that bad." Or worse still: "Be patient. It will pass"

Rather, I say things like, "Yes, the pain in your shoulder may indeed be because of menopause. The good news is it will get better and you probably don't need surgery."

A lot of what I do at the first consultation is reassure a woman that she's actually not going crazy or being "wimpy" and that all the symptoms she has likely have a physiological basis. Sometimes that little piece of information does wonders. Many women tell me they already feel better at the end of the consultation for several reasons: one, they're glad they finally have been able to talk to someone who understands how they feel. Secondly, they are relieved to discover that the problem is not in their heads but is really a physical one. And finally they feel better because they have taken a proactive step in the direction of finding their own cure and relief is at hand.

On that positive note, let's look at some of the symptoms of menopause.

The Scale

In our office we have patients rate all their symptoms on a scale of one to ten, where ten is the worst it could possibly be. Another way to look at it is a gradation of how much of a problem any particular symptom is. You will notice these scales in some of the stories. This gives us a way to monitor a patient subjectively because after all, only the patient knows how she feels.

Symptoms Related to Menopause

General

- weight gain
- hot flashes

- lack of motivation
- fatigue
- insomnia
- underactive thyroid
- low energy
- excess sweating
- vaginal dryness

Psychiatric

- panic attacks
- anxiety
- depression
- decreased sense of self-worth
- mood swings

Neurological

- brain fog
- poor memory
- temperature dysregulation
- off-balance
- dizziness/vertigo
- lightheadedness
- change in vision
- exacerbation of multiple sclerosis

Gastrointestinal

- change in bowel habits
- increased risk of colon cancer
- gas pains and bloating
- sudden bouts of bloating where the waistline increases a couple of inches
- indigestion

Allergies

- new allergies and sensitivities
- hives

Pain

- migraine headaches
- arthritis
- back pain
- muscle cramps
- lowered pain threshold
- shoulder problems

Cardiovascular

- palpitations
- irregular heartbeat
- high cholesterol
- elevated blood pressure

Urinary

- recurrent bladder infections
- cystitis (bladder inflammation)
- frequent urination
- urine leakage with coughing, sneezing, laughter, or orgasm

Musculoskeletal

- rotator cuff problems
- joint pains
- osteoporosis
- muscle aches

Dermatological

- hyperpigmentation
- itching
- blotchy skin
- dry hair, skin, nails
- hair loss or thinning

Connective Tissue

- rotator cuff inflammation
- immune disorders
- arthritis
- tendonitis
- Sjogren's syndrome
- dry eyes

The Brain

The ability of the brain to regulate a variety of functions is very much affected by lack of estrogen. For example, abnormalities in temperature regulation are caused by an area of the brain called the hypothalamus responding to a change in hormone levels. Simply put, the brain's "thermostat" is out of order. This may manifest as hot flashes, but it can also be just a general feeling of being hot all the time or sweating a lot, especially at night.

Hot flashes are the most common symptom of menopause in the Western hemisphere and are presumed to be due to low estrogen levels. So obviously estrogen gets rid of them, but there are other ways to eliminate or reduce them. They usually affect the upper part of the body from the breasts up, but some women get them all over. The typical hot flashes and night sweats are characterized by redness and sweating in the face, neck, and chest. They may be mild but can be debilitating, and external factors can also affect them (for example, drinking hot coffee).

When they occur all over and at night, they are referred to as night sweats. Night sweats tend to last longer than hot flashes; women wake up having soaked their bedclothes, and the frequency of night sweats can cause sleep disturbance. In this way they contribute to fatigue which can interfere with work performance.

> "You should see the look of surprise on my friends' faces when we are talking and realize how similar our nighttime routines are. You should write a chapter called 'The Fan'!"—"Lenda," patient

Poor Sleep

I think lack of sleep is a very underestimated symptom that contributes to a lot of the other problems, such as feeling stressed out, unable to focus, and emotional lability (a term used to describe a tendency to laugh or cry unexpectedly at what might seem the wrong moment and extreme emotional highs and lows). Complaints of low energy and lack of motivation are very common, which may also be related to disordered sleep. Hormonal changes tend to wreak havoc with a woman's sleeping pattern and quality, and this typically causes not just daytime fatigue but a malaise having to do with low energy and often feeling overwhelmed.

Not being able to stay asleep is a common complaint of women going through menopause. Exhausted women go to bed and pass out, only to find themselves wide awake in the early hours of the morning. Poor sleep quality, waking up every three hours, or waking up in the early hours of the morning and not being able to get back to sleep is probably the second most common symptom after hot flashes. Insomnia is no joke. The need for rest is as basic as the need for water and food, and some women have done without sleep for amazing periods of time.

One of my patients told me she had not slept in five years; I was astounded. As a sleep lover, being deprived of sleep would definitely make me crazy.

I often joke when a man complains that his wife is crabby, that we should deprive him of sleep for two weeks straight and then see how functional he would be. After all, sleep deprivation is so bad it has been used as a form of torture.

Unfortunately, because it is so common, this is the symptom that results in a lot of women being given ongoing sleep medication, which leads to several complications like addiction, daytime grogginess, and hazardous driving and exacerbates the problem of lack of focus.

Even with enough sleep some women still complain of severe fatigue. This may be because they lack the motivation to exercise but may also be associated with adrenal fatigue, a condition where the adrenal glands burn out from too much stress. These women cannot get off the couch for more than a few hours and then feel whipped by midafternoon. Adrenal burnout is a result of chronically producing too much cortisol (see chapter 2).

Dryness

Symptoms include dry eyes; dry mouth; itchy, dry skin; vaginal dryness; and dry, brittle hair and nails. Other skin changes include hyperpigmentation (a common, usually harmless condition in which patches of skin become darker in color than the normal surrounding skin); age/dark spots; and excessive hair growth in undesirable places. The skin also may have a loss of firmness and retain fluid in gravity-dependent areas. Thinning hair is a common symptom.

Dryness and thinning of the vaginal lining and genital tissues may lead to painful intercourse and recurrent urinary tract infections. This in turn can contribute to being "turned off" from sexual intercourse.

Weight Gain

This is a major problem for many women, even for those who exercise. The weight gain tends to occur particularly around the middle and occurs at an increased rate in women who have had a hysterectomy. A change in fat distribution and an expanding waistline with perhaps an actual increase in poundage can all be associated with the hormone-deficiency state.

In the breasts, a lot of the glandular tissue is also replaced by fat. Fat at the back of the upper arms and behind the neck is especially associated with unbalanced cortisol levels, which tend to occur in women who have a lot of stress. Around the time of menopause the thyroid can also become sluggish (underactive), which adds to the weight gain and fatigue.

Anxiety

The sudden onset of anxiety symptoms is a classic sign of perimenopause, and sufferers now worry about things they would have considered minor issues before. Women who have always been calm suddenly start to experience panic attacks and claustrophobia.

Panic attacks are anxiety attacks that come on suddenly. They even occur while sleeping and are very scary. Sometimes people who experience a panic attack need to pull over to the side of the road or miss days of work.

Women may make several trips to the ER and get a lot of testing done before they are convinced that "nothing is physically wrong."

Anxiety and panic attacks can be debilitating. Some common symptoms include

- chest pain or a fast heartbeat
- sweating, trembling
- intense terror
- feeling like something terrible is about to happen, or experiencing an altered reality
- the fear that you are going crazy or that you have a severe illness or that death is near
- a smothering, choking sensation
- dizziness, feeling faint, pins and needles in the extremities
- hot and cold flashes

Many women are resigned to taking regular doses of tranquilizers like Xanax and Valium just to remain functional, but if you are inclined to avoid these types of medications, there are other ways to deal with this phenomenon. Bioidentical hormone-replacement therapy (BHRT) is one. Patients who are lucky enough to end up with an experienced therapist may get to bypass all the tranquilizer prescriptions and be sent to get their hormones balanced. It is amazing how many women have spent years taking medication and psychotherapy with minimal improvement and have never been told that their problem is hormonal.

Personality Changes

With menopause there is a lowering of serotonin levels. (Serotonin is an important neurotransmitter that it is associated with feelings of happiness and well-being.) Mood changes and mood swings are another common complaint among women. Not only is it challenging for them, but their mood shifts affect others around them.

We all know someone who seemed to become a completely different person after age forty-five. Whereas she used to be fun to be around and easy to get along with, she is now easily irritated and picky. One patient told me she hates it when her husband says, "You are becoming your mother!" Women in menopause can be unduly nervous or sometimes outright depressed.

I see it all the time in my family medicine practice, someone who has no complaints related to the "change" but just seems so different. A person who previously I couldn't convince to come in even for a physical is suddenly always in the office and very demanding. I notice it more if I haven't seen her for a while because then it seems like a big change. Her family, however, may have been easing into it gradually.

Some women in particular seem to become hypochondriacs. "How do you know it's just a cold?" one lady who called me on a Saturday evening said. "I have an enlarged gland and need an antibiotic called in!"

Women who used to shrug things off must have an appointment *today*! And they never seem to be satisfied. Having been in practice for so long, I can look back and remember how sweet these individuals used to be. Is life just beating them down, or is it their hormones? If I breathe a sigh of relief when they leave the office, I can only imagine what it is like to live with them. Sometimes these women seem to their loved ones (and to themselves) to have become someone else overnight.

The mood swings and emotional lability result in a "Jekyll-and-Hyde-like" personality. They are wound up and irritated by everything and everyone; one such patient told me, "The nicer my husband is to me the more he irritates me and the madder I get!"

This symptom alone can put a lot of stress on the family, coworkers, and friends and of course on the woman herself because she doesn't like being who she has become, yet she feels she can't control it.

Seventy percent of the women I treat have asked themselves at some point if they are "going crazy." They are always relieved to find out that there is a physiological reason for their change in personality.

Women often say, "I just want to be me."

Usually a doctor hearing this instantly moves into the algorithm they are taught in medical school. Their antennae go up, and they wonder if this person has mental-health issues.

The slippery slope toward medication starts. On the other hand, having heard this complaint so many times I know exactly what a woman means when she says this. She is not trying to be a Hollywood celebrity, a sexual dynamo, a glamour queen, or even the life and soul of the party. She just wants to feel like her normal old self, something that is readily achievable.

Depression

An all-too-prevalent psychiatric symptom is depression, which can severely devalue the quality of life for some sufferers. It is very common in perimenopause and postmenopause, as well as episodically in women with PMS.

Once when I was in a psychiatry lecture on depression in medical school I was told about a condition called melancholia, which struck women in their midlife. Melancholia was a term used for middle-aged women who became severely depressed and withdrawn. It was just presented as a fact of life that some women lost themselves when they went through menopause and no one ever mentioned that it was due to or reversible with hormones. The message I got was that it was one of those weird things that happened to middle-aged women sometimes.

It came back to mind recently when one of my patients told me she had just made a stunning discovery. Her grandmother had spent several years in a mental institution after menopause. It was a family secret that was never mentioned until she died. She says all she remembered was that her grandmother was always very quiet and rarely said much at family functions. It is clear to me from the description that this poor lady suffered from melancholia.

She may even have received shock therapy for it in those days. Now facing menopause, my patient had noticed a major alteration in her mood, and she was afraid she would be like her grandmother. (She is currently on bioidentical hormones and doing fine.)

Often in women with a prior history of depression, the doctors assume the patient's medication needs to be increased when the change is really hormonal. In my experience, if the depression got worse with perimenopause, it was likely to improve with hormone treatment. Some patients can actually come off their antidepressants. At the same time, many women are prescribed antidepressants by their doctors just for the treatment of hot flashes.

Neurohormonal Changes

Besides mood changes, the brain is also a critical player in menopause in a different way. The neuroendocrine (hormones that come from the brain itself) changes are fascinating. The relationship between hormones and brain function is well documented in scientific literature [12, 13, 14, 69] Many hormones and neurotransmitters play critical roles in maintaining cognitive (smart power) function in women. The decrease in estrogen and other hormones like melatonin and serotonin affect the brain's ability to process information and multitask, hence the well known "brain fog" that takes over women during PMS and perimenopause and postmenopause.

The common complaint of foggy thinking is where women notice not feeling as mentally sharp as they used to be. This is a major problem, especially for women in jobs that require mental stamina and acuity. The ability to learn and store memory can be impaired. Women have difficulty remembering words, names, and things they knew previously.

NADU A. TUAKLI, MD, MPH

Research studies have shown that estrogen has a neuroprotective effect on the aging brain. Balance problems are common.

Katarina was a forty-eight-year-old woman who started to experience dizziness. She saw a neurologist, an ENT (ears/nose/throat specialist), and various other doctors who couldn't figure out what was wrong. After almost two years of testing they sent her to Johns Hopkins for additional testing then she was told that she had BPPV (benign paroxysmal positional vertigo, a condition that causes a sensation of spinning that occurs suddenly and when the head is turned), which was a harmless condition but she would have to stay on medication indefinitely to control the symptoms.

The medication (meclizine) she was given to control her dizziness made her feel groggy, tired, and confused, which she felt was worse than the dizziness. She decided it was better to deal with her symptoms. One day she heard about bioidentical hormones, and after some research she made an appointment in my office. Once she was started on BHRT, the vertigo and lightheadedness went away.

Multiple Sclerosis

People may develop MS after menopause or relapse from their previously diagnosed condition. It is clear that hormones have an effect on this condition. Pregnancy usually improves it, at least temporarily. (See the chapter on treatment for more on this). Many women with MS are helped by Estrogen therapy. In Europe Estriol (E3) is specifically used for this purpose unfortunately it is not FDA "approved" so many MS patients don't have access to it in the United States.

Pain

Pain can occur anywhere. Musculoskeletal pain is the commonest type. Symptoms are often similar to fibromyalgia, including general muscle achiness, and painful joints (hips and shoulders). It is fairly common to develop rotator cuff tendonitis, which fortunately tends to be temporary and usually resolves with nonsurgical measures. (I developed this condition myself, first in one shoulder and then the next a couple of years later. My colleague offered me arthroscopic surgery to fix it, but I declined. Today my shoulders are both perfectly fine all I needed was a little physical therapy.)

Beware, if you are told you have suddenly developed a rotator cuff problem out of the blue, check your hormones and think long and hard before doing any surgery. Sometimes a woman develops a "frozen" shoulder from a minor shoulder injury that's ignored or improperly treated. Most will resolve with a cortisone shot and physical therapy that is started promptly.

In my experience almost all the women who are diagnosed with "fibromyalgia" or chronic fatigue syndrome are in the perimenopausal/ menopausal age group. The women diagnosed with these conditions probably don't all have the same problem, but it tends to be a catchphrase for women who have symptoms the doctors can't figure out. It is my belief that both conditions are exacerbated by hormone imbalance.

Fortunately most women going through perimenopause and menopause are not incapacitated to such a degree that they get labeled with either of these, but it does happen.

Interestingly, in a Latin American study of 8373 women 90 percent had menopause symptoms, muscle and joint pains and physical and mental exhaustion along with depressive mood were more highly prevalent than hot flashes. Most appeared 5 years before menopause [15].

Many studies from Nigeria also show that muscle and joint pains are the main symptom of menopause (over 80%) along with loss of libido. [16, 17]

Thinning of Bones

Lack of estrogen is a major risk factor for osteoporosis. Other risk factors include having a small frame, Caucasian ancestry, smoking, bulimia, anorexia, low-calcium diet, excessive use of alcohol, and being thin. A family history of osteoporosis is such a significant risk factor that if you have a strong family history, hormone replacement should be a definite consideration.

Heart and Artery Changes

Myocardial infarction (MI; heart attack) and related heart disease are the leading cause of death in men and women over 50 (CDC 2010 data)[19]. It is a complex trait that includes a lot of environmental and genetic factors, but it has been well documented that women have a protective advantage against MI compared to men prior to menopause.

However, various heart issues present themselves during perimenopause and menopause. This is when women lose their protection and their statistics for heart attacks rapidly catch up with their male counterparts. Some factors causing the increased risk of heart disease include increased blood pressure, increased LDL cholesterol, and increased heart rate. Experts believe the hormones that are produced prior to menopause are the key.

Other less harmful heart-related issues include palpitations, which are often reported by perimenopausal women. These may be uncomfortable and worrisome and add to their anxiety.

Incontinence Issues

Some women develop frequent bladder infections particularly associated with intercourse, or they may just have to go to the bathroom many times a day for no apparent reason.

Stress incontinence, where there is some leakage of urine every time a person coughs, laughs, or sneezes, can also be bothersome.

There is a poorly understood condition called interstitial cystitis, where the bladder becomes inflamed for no apparent reason. It causes a lot of pain in some women, and they are usually only diagnosed after many months of pelvic pain and diagnostic testing.

The following is a testimonial from a patient who suffered from this condition.

Testimony of "Evelyn W"

When I went to see Dr. Nadu Tuakli I had already had interstitial cystitis (IC) for a year. I had been seeing an urologist for this condition. According to the urologist IC is permanent, and it is not known what causes it. To best describe what IC is like, I would say the inside lining of my bladder is like a bloodshot eye. Flare-ups are very painful and cause frequent urination. It really can be quite unbearable and debilitating. I had seen the urologist for a number of treatments trying to control the symptoms. These treatments involved being catheterized and having DMSO (dimethyl sulfoxide) pumped into the bladder. After many treatments I was distraught. My urologist said many people opt to have their bladders removed and wear a urostomy bag. At forty-nine, I absolutely did not want to resort to that if I could help it.

My initial visit to see Dr. Tuakli was to discuss adding bioidentical hormones to my daily regimen, and to see how she felt this could benefit me physically and emotionally. I had been experiencing many menopausal symptoms, including IC. Dr. Tuakli went over all these symptoms and questioned me about all aspects of my health, uncovering other areas that she felt she could provide help.

Dr. Tuakli asked if I had ever taken d-mannose (a nutritional supplement). I had never heard of it. She told me it was a supplement of simple sugar and felt that taking this everyday would give me the relief I needed. She went on to recommend other vitamins along with the bioidentical hormones. I was thrilled to have some direction and very thankful for the education she shared with me. My physical and emotional health has definitely improved since I have been a patient of Dr. Tuakli's. The most miraculous part has been that I have not had to return to the urologist for any more treatments, so much better than the alternatives.

There are marked cultural differences in menopausal symptoms in different geographical regions, more than ninety percent of indigenous women in Peru (Quechua) and Colombia (Zenu) at all age intervals had high scores for urogenital symptoms much higher than that described anywhere else in the world. [20]

When your doctor or partner says what ails you probably has nothing to do with your hormones, don't believe it. It almost always does. Menopause affects all women. It doesn't cause life-threatening symptoms, but it can *devastate* a woman's quality of life. Acquiring information gives you the power to understand what is happening to your body, and then you can figure out for yourself the most appropriate path for you. Addressing these symptoms will optimize your well-being.

As for how long the symptoms may last, it varies. Don't hold your breath, one Swedish study showed that women over 85 were still having hot flushes [22].

Action Plan

- You can choose to do nothing about perimenopause or menopause, or you can choose to replace what you have lost.
- Options include replacing them with bioidentically similar hormones, or replacing them with synthetic hormones. Another poor option is to merely treat the individual symptoms with different remedies and/or pharmaceuticals.
- Check your baseline hormone levels *now,* whatever phase you are in.
- Listen to your body and learn more by reading this and other books so you can take charge of your menopause.

MYTH BUSTER ALERT: Despite the fact that it occurs in females, menopause is not a gynecological problem. The ideal person to handle all your symptoms is a family practitioner (shameless plug) who is familiar with all the organ systems.

Unfortunately, more patients are referred to me from a therapist's office than from their gynecologist (See chapter 8).

*

The following highlights a patient with classic perimenopause.

Mary T was at the supermarket, idly looking at all the magazines telling her how to have better sex when she realized that she had *not had sex* in more than a month. *Don't they have other things to do?* she thought.

It wasn't that she and her husband didn't like each other anymore; it was just that life had gotten so busy. He had recently been on a business trip, and she was busy with her practice. Since he got back, it was difficult to find the time and energy to make love. Then again he would probably always find the time and energy, but truth be told she just didn't have the inclination. *When was the last time I really felt horny?* she wondered. With the amount of stress she was under, it was difficult to find time for any self-gratifying activities. *Maybe he hasn't bothered me since he got back because he "got some" while he was away,* she thought. To pursue that line of thought would take too much effort, so she let it go.

She checked her calendar. Work had suddenly become stressful; she and her coworkers used to get along, but now it seemed like it was one problem after the next. She could barely stand to go to work these days; there was so much tension and stress in the atmosphere. Why was everyone so irritating these days?

At this point everything should be so good: she was finished having children and had a successful career, nice house, was settled, and apparently had no worries. Yet she could fly off the handle at the flip of a switch. Sometimes she was just mad at herself for being so mad!

It all came to a crisis point a few months later when she discovered her husband was having an affair.

She decided to embark on a "self-improvement strategy." With hormone balancing, her personal and work relationships improved, and she is finding herself much more fulfilled now. She and her husband are working on their marriage with counseling.

HOW DO YOU SPELL RELIEF?
Freaked out
Burning up
Dried up
Sweaty
Losing it
Brittle bones
Off balance
Bummed out Wits end

Chapter 5

Sexual Intimacy

Erotic love is the spindle on which the earth turns.
—Octavio Paz

S EX IS A complicated subject and is hard to generalize. On the other hand, there are some issues that are common to most women, and addressing these may help gain a better understanding of sexual intimacy in general, including after perimenopause.

Communication and intimacy are known to be the glue of relationships. Because of its sensitive and intimate nature, sex can be a powerful bonding experience between partners. Of course just as there may be love without sex, there may be sex without intimacy. It is difficult to be intimate when you feel irritable and hot.

"You look hot (in that dress)!" may sound like a compliment under thirty-five, but women older than forty-five may not be so sure! It could be construed as a reference to an incipient hot flash.

The discussion of unsatisfying sex in menopause deserves its own chapter because this is an almost universal complaint for women approaching mid-life. Frequently I get questions like: "Is sex supposed to hurt?" "How come I'm just not interested anymore?" "Should I accept that this part is over for me?" Barely a week goes by without someone complaining about her lack of sex drive.

Taking hormones will not necessarily resolve all of a woman's sexual concerns, but hormone balancing can definitely help. There are multiple factors to be taken into account with this complex subject (see below).

It is well known that the two things married couples argue about most are sex and money. Men love sex, and even when they can't physically perform the sexual act, they still crave it. Unfortunately, many *para*menopausal (this includes perimenopausal and postmenopausal) women often do not. Rare is the woman who says, "My sexual relationship has become so much better since I started going through menopause."

Several husbands have confided in me that they think their wives don't "like" them anymore, and as a consequence, they feel less attractive. They take the lack of libido personally when it is simply a biological issue. Marital stress is one of the common problems associated with lack of libido.

Clearly, making babies is not the prime reason most people at any age have sex. More common reasons include expressing love and intimacy to seeking sheer primordial pleasure. But let's look briefly at why nature made it so pleasurable.

In a nutshell, there is a primitive drive across the animal kingdom for this purpose to ensure the propagation of the species. The difference is that with humans, sex has evolved into being an end in and of itself. Intercourse produces feel-good hormones that give us a feeling of nurturing as well as physical and psychological release. For some people, sex is more important than food. A study showed that successful aging was positively associated with self-rated scales of quality of life and sexual satisfaction.[2]

Also, a Taiwanese study showed that people with more sexual activity lived longer. [24]

Another showed mortality risk was 50 percent lower in a group of people with a higher orgasm frequency. [25]

So for a variety of reasons, couples want to stay sexually active—but nature doesn't do much to support or promote it as we mature. And there is often a mismatch in desire between sexual partners.

When a female child is born, her ovaries have more than seven hundred and fifty thousand eggs. Each cycle generates the rupture of one of these eggs from its cyst, which stimulates hormones to be produced.

---

[2] Wesley Thompson, PhD, et al. "Association between Higher Levels of Sexual Function, Activity, and Satisfaction and Self-Rated Successful Aging in Older Postmenopausal Women." *J Am Geriatr Soc.* August 2011; 59(8): 1503–1508. Published online July 28, 2011. doi: 10.1111/j.1532-5415.2011.03495.x.

Beginning at puberty, one egg is released with each ovulation; the rest are gradually absorbed over time. Fewer and fewer eggs remain during perimenopause, and then when they are all gone, the ovaries no longer produce significant amounts of estrogen or progesterone.

At this point, nature decrees that a woman no longer has any need for the sex drive, and her testosterone levels drop and may disappear. Even if she had a high sex drive before, a menopausal woman will experience at least a 40 percent decrease in libido. Why? Because her production of the hormones that control the sex drive has decreased. Thus, women who say they do not notice any difference in their sex drive before and after menopause are either out of touch with their bodies, in denial, or just not telling the truth. Among menopausal women, a change in libido is almost universal—as universal as stopping their periods.

A decrease in libido is normal in a forty-something-year-old woman—just as a decrease in sexual function is normal in a middle-aged man.

Most sexual dysfunction in postmenopausal women is due either to this decrease in interest or to physical difficulties with sexual function. In my experience, the problem tends to lie more with the former. Men are the reverse in this regard. They may not be able to achieve physically what they desire emotionally and psychologically. However, women are living longer and want a more vibrant sex life, and there is a disconnect if the libido is not considered. Many women want to be able to maintain a satisfying relationship with the same level of vitality they had before menopause.

Libido

Even though it may not be the first thing that comes to mind when you think of intercourse, the most important sex organ is the brain for both sexes. The entire sexual experience is affected by what a woman thinks and how she feels about herself and her partner, and there are sociological factors. It is a very complex issue.

Some women find sex more pleasurable because they don't have to worry about getting pregnant, and there may be an empty nest, so a woman has more time to focus on herself and her partner. Also, women generally grow more comfortable with their bodies as they get older.

On the other hand, the desire for sex is obviously a critical component of the sexual relationship, and many women (and their partners) find having a low sex drive to be a major problem.

In a rare minority, the imbalance of hormones causes an increased libido. In some women this can cause even more distress than having none at all, especially with an aging partner. I recently had a patient with this problem. She was very uncomfortable with her increased sexual desire and was relieved to have it restored to normal with hormonal therapy. However, she is an exception to the rule. Libido clearly varies, so one cannot generalize.

Some women felt somewhat indifferent even when they were younger and only had sex when their husbands felt like it. "I don't like it anyway," they may say, overlooking one slight problem: "Your husband *does*!"

Even women with a naturally low libido notice a major difference in their sex drive as their originally low libido disappears and intercourse becomes uncomfortable due to lack of lubrication. Then the discomfort during sex causes apprehension and avoidance, which creates a vicious cycle.

Then a woman who started with little interest in sex initially may come to actively dislike it. This will have an effect on her husband's level of satisfaction as well as her own, and on her marriage. I know of cases where this has been the root cause of some husbands' so-called midlife crisis. Even single women suffer from reduced libido and may lose their desire to masturbate.

Fortunately, one is not stuck with this state of affairs. There are several solutions to improve a libido that has decreased.

What's Culture Got to Do with It?

These scenarios with regard to waning of libido tend to describe American women in particular. In some cultures, women are taught to ignore their libidos altogether.

In many cultures it is not acceptable for a woman to even suggest that she enjoys sex. An extreme example of this is female circumcision, in which the clitoris is removed in an effort to make sure women won't enjoy intercourse.

In these cultures mature women don't complain about loss of libido, probably because they've been trained not to even acknowledge their sexual desires. It is cultural norms like these that tend to reinforce a fear of making changes. Some cultures in West Africa have created a custom in response to the supposed "inevitable" loss of libido. When a woman becomes menopausal, she picks out a younger woman as a "junior wife" for her husband, thus accommodating his sexual needs without having to bother having sex herself.

A friend of mine explained it to me this way: "You know, women of a certain age don't like all that business anymore. She doesn't have to be pestered, but she can still control who her husband is sleeping with."

Well, that's one way to do it. But, needless to say, in many parts of the world this would *not* be an acceptable solution.

I believe menopause presents problems with libido and sex across generations and cultures, issues that women should feel free to discuss without shame.

Remember, if you have no libido, it's no one's fault and you are not to blame. It's just a reality of life, and the sooner you can find ways to accept the reality the sooner you'll be able to take steps to address it and improve your sex life if you choose to.

How Can You Improve Your Libido?

Hormones can help improve your libido. But they won't make you perpetually aroused, if that is not your historical norm. The ideal is for you to be able to return to who you naturally are. (You'll learn more about the hows and whys of hormone supplementation in chapter 6.)

But before you think about taking hormones, it helps to consider some lifestyle changes. First of all, do a stress inventory. Make a list of the stressors in your life. Then, figure out what factors are within your control to change. For example, if you have no unscheduled time for recreation and recharging, your libido will suffer no matter what else you do. Work on adjusting your stress-reaction to certain demands in your life.

Use stress management techniques, avoid alcohol, exercise more, and take B vitamins. Read sexy books or magazines. Review your relationship and seek ways to improve it. A supportive, uncritical partner promotes libido; the opposite suppresses it.

Examine your surroundings. Is your environment conducive to sexual activity? If you have teenagers or your parents in the house, are they cramping your style? How about sending the parents on a cruise with their grandchildren? Designate a regular day of the week for date nights. Consider sex therapy together to help adjust to your new rhythm.

Factors that Affect Function

Physical changes due to lack of estrogen, progesterone, and testosterone can affect your physical functioning irrespective of your interest in intercourse.

These factors include your

- physical health
- medications
- gynecological problems

As you age, lower levels of estrogen decrease the acidity of the vagina, making it more susceptible to infection. The vaginal walls become thinner and less elastic. In some women the vagina actually becomes physically smaller, and there is less lubrication. When the lining cells of the vagina have estrogen, they secrete a natural lubricant; without it they are dry and less flexible.

Your general physical health and well-being affect your sexuality, and vice versa. For example, you are not likely to have satisfying sexual activity if you have pain, are depressed, feel exhausted, can't move in certain ways, or are incontinent.

Having less estrogen long-term also affects the nervous system: women experience decreased sensitivity and responsiveness to touch and vibration. The clitoris and genital area in general may lose sensitivity and may take longer to reach orgasm.

These changes are even more noticeable in longstanding diabetics.

Some medications, including antibiotics, can cause sexual dysfunction in women, which can increase vaginal infections; decongestants and antihistamines can dry the vaginal membranes, and some blood-pressure medication and some antidepressants can make it harder for a woman to achieve orgasm.

Ovarian cysts and other anatomical abnormalities may cause pain; so can urinary-tract infections, interstitial cystitis, and constipation.

Vaginal dryness from decreased lubrication is commonly associated with menopause; however, there are many causes of dryness *not* related to age or menopause that are treatable without estrogen. Never douche or use perfumed vaginal hygiene products. Vaginal dryness may be worse after long periods of abstinence.

Now for the *good news*!

Most research shows that postmenopausal women still have an intact sexual response and they can still have orgasms if they were previously orgasmic. Unlike men, who experience increasing erectile dysfunction with age, women do not have a corresponding *physical* impediment to great sex as they age.

Despite many people's perceptions to the contrary, painful, uncomfortable, and unsatisfying sex does not *have* to be inevitable at any age. People in their eighties are dating, now especially with online dating sites. I was recently told about a lady who is eighty-nine and hadn't had sex for thirty years. She recently became sexually active again with a ninety-two-year-old man. They shared that they both find their intercourse satisfying.

If your sex life is unsatisfactory:

- Adjust your social issues first, and then deal with stress, relationships, and your work/life balance.
- Get a complete physical exam to make sure you don't have any medical issues.
- List what medications you are on and discuss them with your doctor.
- Consider hormone replacement if needed.

Modern society dictates that one must be young in order to be sexy. Folklore and jokes condition us to think so, but before you resign yourself to a sexless existence, consider this: most people are sexually active throughout their lives, particularly if they have a partner. Having an intimate and loving relationship can keep couples indefinitely happy and healthy. Sex can be just as physically and emotionally satisfying in later years as it was before menopause.

Here are two more stories about my patients that show how sexual dysfunction affects women's lives. After each one I have made comments about the case.

Case One

A forty-two-year-old female came in complaining about a physical inability to have sexual intercourse. She said her husband likes sex but she doesn't. This lady's overture began, "I don't really have any *real* menopausal symptoms and only get hot flashes when my husband is in town" (I sensed a fair amount of denial). Luckily for her, her husband travels a lot.

As she warmed up more details began to surface. She said emphatically, "The last time he could not even penetrate because it was too painful and I told him to forget this"

Their marriage had started to feel the strain, and they went to marital counseling at their church. She complained that the counselor was much younger than them and didn't really seem to "get this whole menopause thing. 'Can't you see a doctor?' he asked. Like I have a *medical* condition!" she told me angrily. When she followed his advice and saw a physician, she was given Estrace (a pharmaceutical estradiol) cream.

She said it helped the vaginal dryness but she didn't like using it. "It was messy, and I still didn't like having sex, so what was the point?" After some research she decided to see me for a consultation (she was relieved to find I was a little older than her marriage counselor).

The medical term for pain during intercourse is dyspareunia. Pain is clearly no fun, and it has several causes, one of which may be atrophic vaginitis, a result of menopause. My feeling is that mainly because of this symptom her marriage was on a collision course, yet it was totally rectifiable. I started her on some combination BHRT cream.

She is currently teaching and holding down a second job. She is getting along much better with her husband now. She also notes that in addition to an improvement in sexual function, she is calmer and better able to handle stress. I saw her recently and she was very happy. She said her husband is a "different man". They are planning to travel together on his trips in the summer.

Case Two

Suzie G is a forty-four-year-old who has been complaining of recurrent vaginal infections for a year. She has been having irregular periods for two years but says apart from occasional hot flashes, she was doing okay. She came to see me because she said she was beginning to feel "crazy" from the lack of sleep and night sweats.

"I have been trying to wait this out," she said, "but I'm getting very irritated. How long is this supposed to last?" Apparently "it" was the menopausal transition.

"I know you mentioned hormones, but I kind of like not having my period all the time." A deeper discussion revealed a common misconception; she associated going on hormones with the recurrence of monthly periods. I asked if her not wanting to have periods had something to do with sexual activity, but then she dropped a major bombshell.

"Oh no!" she said. "There's nothing going on in the sex department. It's just so uncomfortable. I don't enjoy it. We tried lubricating jellies, but they don't help. At least when I have a vaginal infection I have an excuse. I never dreamed I would be giving up sex at this age."

While I'm not trained as a psychotherapist, it occurred to me that this patient's emotions surrounding sex and intimacy might very well be causing her a great deal of stress. Stress can compromise the immune system, opening the door to a variety of illnesses, including yeast infections.

She then echoed a sentiment that I hear from many women. "I feel sorry for my husband. He keeps bugging me and then I finally give in, but it's like okay, hurry up and get done. He knows I'm not interested, but he's so desperate he's happy to take it."

She said that for two years I had been "hinting" that hormones might help, and in the meantime things had gone from bad to worse. "Do you have something herbal I can take to solve this problem?"

"Why are you reluctant to try hormones?" I asked. "You are forty-four and have given up sex?"

"Well, I want to tough it out."

"At what cost? So you can say you did it the hard way?"

I find this case interesting because it shows many common misconceptions. First, why is it necessary to "tough it out"? There are no medals to be won for suffering. Secondly, hormones do not necessarily bring back your periods. In fact, you don't have to have your periods at all.

Thirdly, misinformation is causing this young lady to put her marriage in peril. She feels like she's going crazy; she's fatigued, and her work performance is going downhill just so she can say, "At least I didn't take hormones"!

On the other hand she's happy to take anything that might be classified as *herbal,* even if it's not as effective. I gave her high doses of probiotics to reduce the recurrence of her yeast infections.

Apparently she took my desire to remain objective as "hinting." I don't push hormones on anyone because I believe it's a personal choice. I merely proffer information. Every woman needs to weigh the pros and cons of her situation and do what she feels is best for herself and her relationship.

Chapter 6

Treatment of Menopause

"Replace what is missing"
—Dr. Nadu Tuakli

CAN YOU REPLACE deficient hormones? What are bioidentical hormones? Are they natural? Do they cause cancer? Why are they controversial? What are compounding pharmacies, and how are they different from my local supermarket pharmacy?

All of these questions will be answered in this chapter.

My many years in practice taught me that if you give patients medical information in a clear, concise, and uncluttered fashion, they get it! Which is the point of this book.

Here's the deal: if you don't think you feel optimum, you deserve to feel better. Seek out the solution—demand it.

There is a common tendency to ignore problems with the philosophy of "if it ain't broke, don't fix it." This is not necessarily a good policy when it comes to your health. Here we try to catch things before they are broken, not wait around until they deteriorate.

I definitely do not want to give the impression that women need to be "fixed," since perimenopause and postmenopause are normal phases of life, not illnesses. However, it's important to acknowledge that some individuals need more help than others—while there are some people who feel they need no help at all. "To each her own"

The menopause syndrome is a treatable phenomena, and the way in which it is handled is a matter of personal preference.

In my experience, women almost always have more to gain than they have to lose by taking hormones, but it is not for me to make that choice for them. I give suggestions, including sometimes advising women they are on medications they don't need.

Biologically identical hormones are derived from plants like the wild yam or soybean plant. The molecules of the wild yam can be converted in the laboratory to estrogen and other hormones that have a chemical structure the same as those produced naturally in the human body.

Making the Case for Treating Menopause

Menopause is a condition that often needs to be treated because of the profound misery it can cause. Even for those who are *not* miserable, remember the World Health Organization definition of health as "a state of complete physical, mental, and social well-being."

There may be a spectrum of issues, and some may have mild symptoms that can be ignored while others can be so destabilized that it cripples their ability to function.

There are also some who feel that it is their moral duty to grin and bear it regardless of how bad their symptoms are. (Remember, there are no medals!) Women may end up being overmedicated, which only makes symptoms worse. Their quality of life goes rapidly downhill and oftentimes ends up in a midlife crisis or the loss of a job, partner, or self-esteem.

Some women's lives are completely turned upside down. They feel marginalized and disrespected because the medical community does not really appreciate what they are going through. One patient complained to me how belittled she felt when she told her doctor that she thought her inability to lose weight was hormone related. "Now, now, Betty," she was told. "We would all like to be a size five, but unfortunately, as we get older …"

Women's roles in society have drastically changed. The Federal Reserve is now governed by a woman, and we may soon have a female president. It is inconceivable that these women would have this much responsibility and not be able to have their menopausal symptoms handled efficiently, or be overmedicated as they make world-altering decisions! As a physician, I can tell you that I am more able to help others when I myself am in balance.

It's hard to fan yourself and pay attention to a patient at the same time!

If you have determined that you need relief of your menopausal and perimenopausal symptoms, reach out and find it. It's not going to come looking for you. Old-fashioned ideas, pride, misunderstandings, and miscommunications will not be helpful. Avail yourself without fear of what is readily available.

> At the end of the day, women who are challenged by menopause are basically struggling to maintain their quality of life. They have responsibilities, they are contributing members of society, and they also have leadership roles, even if that role is only within the household. Remember, menopause is always treatable.

When a new patient begins by saying, "I don't really know why I am here" (sounds like guilt and shame to me), or "I really should be able to handle this myself ..." (embarrassment and bravado), my first job is to reassure them they are wise for pursuing their options. Knowledge is power.

Does a Hormone Imbalance in a Woman Affect a Man?

Let's not forget that males are often the other half of the bioidentical hormone-replacement story. As with many other things, it is better to take a holistic approach to solving issues. Men generally suffer quietly through their wives' perimenopause, but they suffer nonetheless. Part of that suffering may be because whereas they used to understand their wives, they now find themselves in a position where they do not understand what is going on. This is often a source of stress, including the marital stress that comes from a lack of physical intimacy and pleasure and the uncertainty of knowing "which wife" is going to wake up beside him in the morning. Some men say they feel they have to tip-toe around their spouses because little things set them off.

Because the children are affected, they may avoid their mother as much as possible, and that puts more pressure on the dad to bring up the rear and fill in for the things mom used to do.

One of my patients told me a cute story. She had not realized how her perimenopause was affecting her family until after she started her hormone therapy. She said her nine-year-old son would come running up to the car when she was leaving for work and say, "Mom, did you remember to take your medicine?"

The menopausal syndrome extends beyond the family because it also affects one's coworkers and other members of one's social circle.

How Is Menopause Treated?

Unfortunately, in our culture of instant gratification, people want immediate cures. The result is that many menopausal women are being treated with multiple medications for symptom relief, but this may not be the best thing for them.

My inclination is toward replacing what is missing in as natural a manner as possible. By doing so, potential side effects are minimized, and the body is encouraged to work with what it is most familiar.

This is why I recommend compounded bioidentical hormones. Even when the pharmaceutical companies claim their product is bioidentical, they have patented formulas for the binder, dye, preservative, filler, or adhesive. One of my patients discovered that one contained peanut oil, and she is allergic to peanuts.

Over the years I have seen that postmenopausal women on hormones look better, feel better, and are more active than their counterparts. Because they are more motivated to exercise, it creates a positive cycle. Their brains function better, which leads to an overall improvement in job performance, quality of life, and sense of well-being.

Hormones ease menopausal symptoms; this is a statement of fact. Hundreds of studies have shown that hormones are the most effective way to cure menopausal symptoms. Even so, they are not a panacea, but they *can* help you remake your life and get back to feeling good and positive about the future.

I want women to be aware of the possibilities hormones can create for harmony and balance. Bioidentical hormone-replacement therapy (BHRT) is safe and effective; despite this, misconceptions and unwarranted fears cause millions of women to not benefit from them (see chapter 1). You only need to take the hormone you are deficient in (for example, not everyone needs estrogen).

Some herbs and supplements may work for specific symptoms and can be especially helpful for women who cannot or choose not to take hormones for a variety of reasons. However, for the most part they are band-aids that don't directly address the problem.

There are also other prescription remedies available. In my general medical practice, I have often prescribed antidepressants, particularly a group of medications called SSRIs (selective serotonin reuptake inhibitors), and I have seen them do wonders for depressed women of various ages. Millions of women are living normal lives because of them. I believe that when appropriate, they are very helpful medications. Unfortunately they have also become very socially acceptable, so patients desperate for symptom relief will readily take them for menopause when suggested by their doctors.

Jane's Story: Enough Herbs to Break a Sweat

When I first met Jane she was 47 years old she told me she was having (quote) 'horrible perimenopause'. She had been married for 21 years and smoked ¼ pack of cigarettes per day. She had been reading about perimenopause and had decided to take matters into her own hands.

Depression and anxiety, dry eye, dry lips, itching on the bottom of her feet and in the middle of her back were major problems for her. She couldn't sleep and was having severe panic attacks. She had no libido and was very gassy, you can see her other complaints in the table below.

I was literally amazed at how many pills she was taking, you can see her list below. She said she had come up with her own concoction from reading which helped a little with some specific symptoms. She took her pills diligently trying to feel better. In addition to the herbal supplements and vitamins she was also on Clonazepam (a tranquilizer) for sleep and anxiety. After her consultation with me she decided to try BHRT.

We signed an agreement to stop smoking and got a saliva test which showed that she was low in estrogen, progesterone and DHEA. After I started her on BHRT she gradually tapered off of all her supplements. It took 2 months before she felt completely comfortable letting go of them all.

The symptom profile shows her progress. She is 50 now and doing very well on nothing else besides her hormones.

Jane is one of many women who present with anxiety and panic attacks but one thing that made her unique was the quantity of pills she was taking trying to feel better, unfortunately all to no avail. Interestingly enough when her therapist was discussing Jane with her supervisor she immediately recognized the problem and told her to send her to me rather than a psychiatrist. Clearly, her therapist has a very experienced supervisor, all the therapy (and pills) in the world would not have made her better.

These are the supplements that she was taking before starting BHRT:

Flax Seed Oil liquid
Maca
Evening Primrose
Vitamin D3
Vitamin Bcomplex
Vitamin B6 50 mg twice a day
Zinc 50mg daily
Vitamin E 400 i.u
Magnesium oxide 500mg
Magnesium Glycinate 360mg
Theanine 200mg
Homeopathic formula#9
Homeopathic formula #6
Acacia fiber
Flax Seed fiber
Probiotics
Enzymes
Licorice
"Estro Soy Plus"
Black Cohosh 40mg

NADU A. TUAKLI, MD, MPH

Red Clover 300mg
Vitamin C (Ester-C) 1500mg
5 HTP 100mg in the AM
(For sleep)
"Homeopathic Calm Forte"
Avena
Passion Flower
Clonazepam (RX) 0.25mg at night

Symptom profile for Jane
"Enough herbs to break a sweat"

SYMPTOM	Baseline with herbs	One month with BHRT	Six months later	1 year later	2 years later
Fatigue	6	6	4	3	2
Energy	5	4	2	2	2
Sleep Quality	5	4	2	2	2
Libido	10	10	6	5	7
Depression	5	1	1	1	1
Mood swings	5	3	3	3	2
Hot flashes	7	3	2	2	1
Itchy skin	6	5	2	2	2
Memory	5	5	4	3	2
Dry eyes, lips	5	2	2	2	3
Stress	7	7	5	5	4
Panic/Anxiety	8	4	2	2	2
Exercise	5	5	4	4	2
Overall Wellbeing	6	3	4	4	2

Some people say they don't take bioidentical hormones because their insurance doesn't cover it, but they will pay for antidepressants. Really? Is that what governs how you manage your health?

Mental Health

I think hormone therapy is particularly underrated and underutilized when it comes to mental-health symptoms. Every woman who develops anxiety and panic attacks during the perimenopausal years has relief of these symptoms when her hormones become balanced. This is a far better solution than indefinitely taking tranquilizers. Xanax-like drugs are a dangerous band-aid that lead to developing tolerance and addiction. And when anxiety is due to hormonal deficiency, all the counseling in the world is not going to address the problem.

If you have suddenly developed panic attacks in your perimenopausal years with no prior history of anxiety, *hormone therapy can fix it.* Depression is a common symptom that occurs around middle age and is clearly related to a variety of hormonal imbalances. When a middle-aged woman who has never suffered from depression before all of a sudden feels depressed, it is often because her hormones are malfunctioning.

Although hormones will not cure genetically acquired depression, they can still help with this condition if there is a sudden worsening around the time of menopause. In my opinion, just as with the case of anxiety, any woman who has a new onset of mental disturbances around the time of menopause should try hormones before trying other drugs, to see if they make any difference.

The problem here is that you may use a "band-aid" like an antidepressant to cover the basic problem, and this particular band-aid has multiple side effects, including suppressing your libido, potentiating suicidal thoughts, and accelerating bone loss. Other side effects of antidepressants include weight gain, increased BP, risk of stroke, foggy thinking, and lethargy—all problems you can get with menopause anyway.

Researchers from the University of Massachusetts and Harvard University even found thirty articles associating SSRI antidepressants with an increased risk of breast and ovarian cancers.

Perhaps your responsibilities have increased at work, the kids are know-it-all pains in the rear, you're paying off your mortgage, and you may be responsible for aging parents. These are common stressors, and you need to deal with them as well as take care of yourself.

Hormones can help you focus, lighten the depression, and remove anxiety so you are able to handle these stressful situations and more.

In the chapter on hormones, I explained that estrogen affects mood by influencing neurotransmitters in the brain. One of the neurotransmitters that is increased is called serotonin. Increased levels of serotonin are associated with positive feelings and have a calming effect. Low serotonin levels can be caused by low estrogen, problems with the receptors, or low production. Estrogen receptors are prominent in the brain, the breasts, and the genital system, so these are areas that are particularly responsive to the hormones.

Insomnia

Could you use a good night's sleep?

Hormones will enhance your sleep. Unlike sleeping pills, they are not addictive. If chronic insomnia is interfering with your life and you find that you have been taking sleeping pills for several months, think about taking BHRT. Your sleep pattern will return to normal, and they don't leave you hung over or with mood changes the next day, the way sleeping aids can.

Bladder Problems

Some women get frequent urinary tract infections (UTIs) and bladder problems after menopause (see chapter 4). This is due to changes in the lining of the uro-genital organs from lack of estrogen. Estriol (E3) vaginal cream was studied in women who had recurrent urinary tract infections. In that study, those who used the cream had a major reduction in UTIs from 0.5 per year compared to 5.9 per year in the placebo group. The vaginal pH (acidity) also decreased to healthier levels while there was no change in the placebo group.

The effect of the cream on the uterine lining was also studied, and there was absolutely no thickening compared to the group without the hormone, showing that there was no increased risk of endometrial cancer from using estriol cream.

Arthritis

Like any other machine, if a body keeps moving it can continue to move. When it stays stagnant, the joints (metaphorically) rust. In the United

States, arthritis is the leading cause of joint pain and degeneration. Because women on hormones tend to feel good, they are more likely to stay active, which is good for their weight and their arthritis.

Prevention of Heart Disease

If you have a family history of heart disease, you would be well advised to consider BHRT. Despite the flaws in the studies (see chapter 7 for information regarding WHI, and PEPI studies), progesterone has been shown to be beneficial in improving the lipid (cholesterol) profile. Natural progesterone improves it better than the synthetic medroxyprogesterone (Provera) with fewer reported side effects.

Estrogen improves the lipid profile and also protects against coronary vasospasm. Sometimes a heart attack is caused not by a clot or hardening but by a spasm in an artery (vasospasm). The end result is the same because blood can't get through the artery and so the heart muscle is deprived of oxygen.

Osteoporosis

Good news! Everyone agrees that estrogen is good for the bones. In addition to relieving vasomotor symptoms (e.g., hot flashes) and improving the lipid profile, estrogen helps maintain bone strength. It is mainly E2 (estradiol) that has an effect on bone density. The FDA says prevention of osteoporosis should not be the sole reason to use hormones, but if you have a strong family history of it or develop it prior to menopause, I beg to differ.

For good health estrogen and progesterone should be balanced whether or not a woman has a uterus.

In a Nutshell

Almost all the symptoms discussed in chapter 4 can be eliminated with bioidentical hormones. Here's a quick recap:

- Hormones are great for reducing migraines.
- They can control anxiety, depression, and irritability.
- They can relieve hot flashes and night sweats.
- They can improve one's ability to focus.
- They can promote sound sleep.
- They can enhance your libido.
- They can restore your zest for life.

> The decision to take hormones should be based on your health, on what your symptoms are, and on what your risk factors might be.

Bioidentical Hormone Therapy (BHRT), a More Natural Form of Hormone Replacement

The goal of hormone replacement is to replace deficiencies and create balance using hormones that are biochemically the same as the hormones your own organs made. For the women that say "I just want to be me" this is something that is readily achievable. It is possible for a woman to feel just like her normal self.

Even though I practice anti-aging medicine, no one has ever said to me, "Give me hormones because I don't want to get old"!

To understand what bioidentical means, here is an easy example. Take salt from the sea and distill it, take ordinary table salt and put it on the same plate, and then take sodium and chloride and combine them in a biochemistry lab to make salt. You will then have three samples of salt from three different sources, yet they all taste the same, look the same, and in fact biochemically cannot be differentiated. They are essentially bioidentical.

That's what happens when a compounding pharmacist prepares a bioidentical compound. It's not only made to mimic the natural product, it actually *is* the natural product. So bioidentical estrogen and progesterone that are compounded from plant sources are chemically the same as what is naturally made in the human body. These hormones are made by pharmacists who have special training in compounding. They are customized for the individual patient and are the most natural form of hormone replacement for both men and women. Bioidentical hormones are plant-based but biochemically identical to those made by the human ovaries.

On the other hand, when you look at Premarin and Provera, they are not naturally found in humans. Premarin is bioidentical to horses' estrogen, and Provera is not even found in nature. Nor are any of the components in birth-control pills.

Foreign substances in the body do not make for a harmonious existence. Hormones work in concert, like an orchestra. Each hormone plays its part to keep the body working smoothly like the magnificent machine it is. When you clog it up with less-than-optimal products, it is likely to respond the same way your car does.

Be aware that not all "bioidenticals" are created equal. Pharmaceuticals have co-opted the term, but even though their product may have a bioidentical base, they are not the same as the pure hormones that are compounded. The pharmaceuticals have patented formulas for the preservatives, dyes, and fillers that they use, and in the case of patches, the adhesive. In addition, they only contain estradiol and no estriol, which is the wonderfully protective estrogen.

How Do I Take BHRT?

BHRT can be made into whatever form the patient chooses, and all the necessary hormones can be compounded into one preparation. They can be made into drops, suppositories, patches, injections, pellets, creams, or lozenges, whichever the patient prefers. Ninety-nine percent of my patients take their compounds twice a day by cream, troches, or sublinguals (lozenges that dissolve in the mouth). When used as a cream it is used morning and night on the thin skin inside the wrist or elbow.

One form I do *not* recommend is capsules. Here's why:

Everything ingested by mouth goes into the stomach. Then everything in the stomach is sent by a special vein called the portal system, to the liver. The liver is the main detoxification organ of the body. It is designed this way as a safety mechanism to limit the body's toxic exposure. Once the ingested substance has been detoxified, it is released into the main blood supply and allowed to course around the body.

There are a few reasons you don't want your liver to process your hormones. One is that your liver already has a lot of work to do detoxifying all the other things you take by mouth (e.g., painkillers and alcohol). We know your BHRT compound is safe, so there is no need for it to add to the work of the liver by being detoxified.

Secondly, various protein-clotting factors are made in the liver, and it is known that estrogen and testosterone can cause an increase in these clotting factors. This is thought to be one of the mechanisms by which the birth-control pill increases the risk of blood clots. This risk increases with age and is higher with smokers. (In spite of this well-established fact, millions of women in their forties still take an oral birth-control pill).

Actually, the comparison of the oral contraceptive pill and bioidentical hormone therapy is a good one. One is a completely synthetic compound made from artificial estrogen and progesterone-like hormones. They are taken by mouth and cause a myriad of side effects. The other is similar to that made by the body itself and bypasses the stomach (because it is not a pill) and has much fewer side effects.

The Politics of Hormone Therapy

Giving women hormonal pills is big business. It may not be good for *their* health, but it is certainly good for the economy. Choosing a safer alternative apparently is not.

The use of bioidentical hormones is obviously a subject of intense debate. Almost everyone agrees on the symptoms of menopause (see chapter 4) and the fact that estrogen and progesterone supplementation will relieve all of them. Unfortunately, that is where opinions diverge.

I believe the only reason BHRT is controversial is because the drug companies cannot patent the products and therefore cannot make any money from them. If "Big Pharma" was not involved in dictating what women should do with their lives, there would be a lot less controversy. Why do they care? It is about money. Drug companies spend a lot of money trying to demonize bioidentical hormones. Compounding pharmacies in particular, have been highly maligned.

Billions of dollars per year are made from the millions of women who are becoming menopausal daily. Bioidentical hormones are natural products made from plants, so they cannot be patented (it's like someone trying to patent salt). Without a patent the drug companies cannot have exclusive rights to the drug and cannot make money from it because everyone else can make it too. So what do they do? They spend millions of dollars discrediting the pharmacies that make them and lobby the FDA for them to not be approved. They bully the insurance companies into not paying for them and use scare tactics to make patients and doctors think they are dangerous.

Many doctors worldwide are so programmed that they will only prescribe pharmaceuticals and don't want to take the time to learn about safer alternatives. As a result, many women are denied the benefit of choice.

Compounded bioidentical hormone therapy

- is precisely dosed
- is customized
- is effective
- is economical
- has minimal side effects

Let's look at the hormones used in BHRT prescriptions.

Estrogen

As we discussed in chapter 2, there are three main kinds of estrogen: E1, E2, and E3. A compound that has all three in it is called Triest (triestrogen), and one that only has E2 and E3 is called Biest. Most doctors these days prescribe Biest mainly to mitigate the fear people have that E1 can stimulate any existing breast cancer. Also, because E3 is such a protective estrogen, the Biest has more of it than estradiol (E2). The pharmaceutical preparations of estrogen only contain E2.

Estrogen must always be balanced by progesterone, and it's not only the hard numbers that are important. The ratio between the two is also very important.

Sometimes patients are given estrogen just because they have some symptoms of menopause, yet their problem is not that they don't have enough estrogen, it's that they don't have enough progesterone to balance the estrogen that they do have.

Picture this scenario. A patient with too little progesterone complains of menopausal symptoms to her doctor and is given estrogen. Sometime later she goes back to the doctor complaining of feeling worse. The doctor may think the patient needs more estrogen and keeps adding more, which will make the "estrogen dominance" worse. Too much estrogen as well as too little can cause a person to feel unwell. When the body is out of balance for whatever reason, the person is not going to feel good.

The yin and the yang must balance each other. A common cause of imbalance in the menopausal woman's body stems from the theory that if you don't have a uterus, you don't need progesterone because you can't get uterine cancer. So doctors prescribe estrogen alone even though estrogen by itself (unopposed) can cause problems in other parts of the body. Plus, by itself estrogen doesn't necessarily do the job. Estrogen and progesterone must be balanced for good health regardless of whether you have a uterus.

Unopposed (unbalanced) estrogen is not a good thing for the breasts or the uterus.

Estriol (E3) has been shown to actually *suppress* the growth of some cancerous breast tissue.

Even women who have had breast cancer can use the so-called "safest estrogen" estriol (E3) vaginally. Vaginal estrogen is not absorbed by the body to the same extent as estrogen taken by other routes so has few if any side effects. But if you are taking hormones via another method, it is not usually necessary to use vaginal estrogen as well unless vaginal dryness is still a problem even with systemic hormones.

Progesterone

Remember, do not confuse *progesterone* with progestins. There are different kinds of progestins such as medroxyprogesterone, Provera, or norethindrone, plus a variety of different versions that are used in birth control pills. (See table in chapter 2.) The problem with these progestins is that they actually are not progesterone, and some of them, instead of doing good things the way natural progesterone does, can be detrimental [37].

The highly touted Women's Health Initiative Study (see chapter 7) that was done in 2002 showed that Provera significantly raised the risk of getting breast cancer. But Provera is a progesterone-like substance that was being given to women as a substitute for real progesterone.

Depo-Provera, which is the same compound as Provera, is a commonly used contraceptive. It has been shown to thin the bones, causing osteoporosis in women who use it for many years. Real progesterone does not do this. It is actually beneficial to the bones.

Testosterone

This is another bioidentical hormone that is commonly given to postmenopausal women. It is good for the brain (memory), bones, muscles, and libido in addition to being important with lubrication, energy, and a reinforcing sense of desirability and overall well-being.

Testosterone is not effective if a woman is lacking estrogen and progesterone. Testosterone does have some side effects (most notably increased facial hair, male-pattern baldness, acne, and lowering of the voice, which tends to imply that the dose of testosterone is too high for that individual). The doses given to women usually are too low to cause any of these, but if a women has side effects, she just needs to stop using the testosterone or lower the dose. Testosterone should *never* be taken by mouth because it can cause liver toxicity and affect clotting factors. Fortunately, bioidentical hormones are always given in a way that bypasses the stomach.

Testosterone can also decrease cholesterol and increase the red blood cell count, which is why it used to be given to people with anemia from kidney disease, to help them make more blood.

Treating Libido with Testosterone

Testosterone is the main hormone related to libido but it is not the only one. Most people take testosterone daily, but some women like to just apply it when needed to the genital area an hour before intercourse for arousal purposes.

DHEA, estrogen, and progesterone may all help revive a woman's sex drive.

The medications used for erectile dysfunction in men (such as Viagra) have not been shown to be particularly helpful in women, even though they can increase blood supply to the pelvic area.

In my experience at least 60 percent of women reported an improvement in their libido from using testosterone. But as discussed previously, this is only one of the factors in a complicated issue.

Testosterone is not a panacea and cannot work on its own. It is not going to change sexual dysfunction that existed before menopause and that is unrelated to hormonal issues. On the other hand, sexual intimacy increases your health and that of your relationship. If you had a great sex life before menopause, it can be rekindled with BHRT. For those women who didn't enjoy sex before, help in the form of sex therapy may be helpful.

In addition to the major steroid sex hormones, other hormones can be replaced (see chapter 2)

Is It Natural?

How is natural defined? A lot of people use the term to imply that natural equates to more primitive and inherently safer, yet there are many things in nature that are powerful agents with potential side effects. Arsenic is natural but lethal. So is an excessive intake of salt or even water. So natural is not a particularly helpful word these days, especially because it is not a regulated term in the way organic is.

I commonly hear women say they think they should go through menopause "naturally." What could be more natural than replacing exactly what your body is deficient in? One could consider arthritis and degeneration as being natural, but most people choose not to succumb to it. Nor do they find it unnatural to take medication to improve the symptoms and relieve the pain.

When your skin is dry you put a moisturizer on it to help the texture and relieve the dryness. You don't say, "Well, my skin is naturally dry, and I'm just going to leave it alone to itch, peel, and look ashy." Furthermore, it is natural for humans to ingest what they cannot make themselves. That's why if we can't get enough in our food we take vitamins because the body doesn't naturally make some of them.

With the booming industry of Botox and fillers and the "sixty is the new forty" mindset, the flourishing industry of anti-aging has resulted in the desire to maintain youth. However searching for external youth while rejecting the notion of internal vitality does not make sense—certainly not when what's being ignored is something as basic as a hormone deficiency. The single most effective thing you can do to maintain a vibrant midlife passage is manage your hormones with plant based bioidentical hormones.

Anita's Story : Don't quit your day job

Anita was a lady in her 60's who did not like taking medicine, she always preferred to try natural remedies and she exercised regularly.

Anita had been complaining about her job for years. Her work environment was very stressful and she could not stand her co-workers. I tried to listen empathetically and recommended stress management techniques, I also expressed concern about her rising blood pressure but it fell on deaf ears. After a couple of years she began to have severe hot flashes which she found especially embarrassing at work. Finally it all came to a head, she told me she had been trying to hold out until she could officially retire at 66 but she couldn't take it anymore. She didn't feel that she could handle the stress of dealing with her coworkers for one more day.

I asked her to take a deep breath and a step back. She had just turned 65 was it really worth giving up everything so impulsively? "Get your hormones balanced and if you still feel the same way in 3 months then consider quitting your job. You've worked so hard for so long you deserve your retirement benefits" I told her.

Out of respect for our 17 year relationship she agreed to give BHRT a try. She began to get along much better at work and she told me that even though the situation was essentially the same she was able to handle it and not get stressed.

Her symptom profile is shown below.

Symptom Profile for Anita "Don't Quit your day job"

SYMPTOM	Start (65 y/o)	One month later	One Year later (66)	Two years later (67)
Fatigue	5	2	4	2
Quality of sleep	8	1	4	4
Energy	5	2	4	2
Hot Flashes	7	2	1	1
Libido	5	2	2	2
Depression	3	2	2	2
Mood swings	10	5	2	2
Memory	5	2	5	3
Stress	10	5	10	5
Overall well being	5	2	4	2

Last December at 67 she retired, she stays in touch with her ex-coworkers and she is still doing well on her hormones. We still joke about how I stopped her from shooting herself in the foot and doing something she would have regretted forever.

But Is it Safe?

Side effects

There are potential side effects for everything you put into your system. Salt, aspirin, coffee, cough syrup, and hormones are no exception. Too much of anything is bad, even something as innocuous as water. This is why people on hormones are monitored to make sure their levels are not higher than normal (your symptoms will show if your dose is insufficient). The side effects of hormones tend to be relatively minor when compared to most of the standard medications for conditions like cholesterol, diabetes, hypertension, and erectile dysfunction (which are the top sellers) [39].

There is *no* evidence that bioidentical hormones actually cause cancer. As an extra preventive measure there have been some calls in the medical community for universal testing for the genetic mutations that cause ovarian and breast cancer in women older than thirty. The idea is to be able to pick out those who are at increased risk. It may also reduce the worry for some people about developing breast cancer, even though fewer than 5 percent of breast cancers are hereditary.

Depending on the hormone, there can be some unwanted side effects.

- Estrogen may cause breast tenderness, irregular bleeding, and excessive thickening of the endometrium (uterine lining), which theoretically can lead to uterine cancer if unchecked, although there are no studies that confirm this.
- Progesterone may cause water retention and sleepiness.
- Testosterone may be responsible for acne, facial hair growth, and hair loss.
- DHEA can contribute to acne.

NADU A. TUAKLI, MD, MPH

Usually the side effects are dose dependent, so you can reduce the dose and they go away. Life-threatening side effects are rarely reported (see studies in chapter 7).

Getting Started on Treatment

You should always start any treatment in consultation with your doctor, of course—but before visiting the doctor, your first duty is to educate yourself so you know what questions to ask.

Who is a candidate for BHRT?

Any woman who needs relief of menopausal symptoms and does not have any medical condition that precludes her from taking them (for example, smokers; a woman with active hormone responsive cancers like breast and ovarian; a woman with a history of heart disease or multiple risk factors for developing it; a woman with a personal or family history of blood clotting problems or conditions that put her at increased risk such as morbid obesity) is a viable candidate.

Which women may want to strongly consider BHRT?

- women who don't have the above exclusions and who have menopausal symptoms that are impacting their quality of life
- women who have severe PMS and or perimenopause
- women with a strong family history of severe osteoporosis
- middle-aged women who are suffering recent onset of anxiety and/or depression

A patient of mine hadn't had a pap smear for eight years because it was just too uncomfortable for her to bear; this could be dangerous. Now, on BHRT, she gets her test regularly and complains that the insurance company wont pay for her to have one annually!

How much do they cost?

Hormones cost starts at about $30 to $40 a month, probably less than getting your hair or nails done. The cheapest form of the hormones is the cream form. Up until January this year insurance companies were paying a portion of the prescription but as the drug company lobby expands its influence less and less companies will cover it. Sometimes you can get them to cover separate components such as estradiol, testosterone or progesterone cream and then you would have to pay for a separate prescription of Estriol which is inconvenient but may circumvent the insurance refusing to pay. Work it out with your doctor and pharmacist to see what is most cost effective. Lobby your insurance company and your employer to get it paid for.

What is the prescription?

BHRT is very individualized and the prescription is customized to a particular patient. The prescription is usually given morning and night because the hormones last about 12 hours.

All patients are carefully monitored and should feel confident that they are doing something to enhance not detract from their health.

When your cortisol level is normal, thyroid is optimal, testosterone, progesterone and estrogen are balanced, you will feel back to 100 percent. Yes, happy and excited about the future.

> *It's up to you take charge of your menopause!*

A Testimonial from an MS Patient

I was touched to receive the following testimonial from one of my patients, in which she describes her struggle with hormonal changes during menopause:

NADU A. TUAKLI, MD, MPH

A number of years ago, as I was immersed in the throes of menopause, I happened upon a book about treating menopausal symptoms with bioidentical hormones. Standing in the bookstore and leafing through the book, I found it described the myriad of symptoms I was experiencing at the time: frequent intense hot flashes; fitful sleep patterns marked by waking up drenched with sweat every night; moodiness and irritability; forgetfulness; fluctuating dry, itchy skin to clammy skin; and last but not least, a plummeting libido! Adding further insult to injury, after I had described my symptoms to my family practitioner and my gynecologist, they both thought I was depressed and wanted to prescribe an antidepressant. I told them I was not depressed, said no to the antidepressant, and walked out of their offices silently fuming! I was especially disappointed that my female gynecologist did not take me more seriously.

Interestingly enough, I do not remember my mother having many complaints during her "transition" other than that she would occasionally get flushed and state she was having a hot flash. Therefore, I never really considered menopause to be a problem and thought I would "transition" seamlessly, as she did.

Unfortunately, that was not the case. As a practicing registered nurse, an artist, a wife, a mother, and a grandmother, I felt I could no longer completely function in any area of my busy life. I was getting more and more overwhelmed. I was continually exhausted from the lack of sleep, and the forgetfulness was a constant fear, especially for someone who in the past was able to think and act quickly on her feet. It was all I could do to drag my exhausted body home and then face making dinner and doing all the other chores that are just a part of life. My husband had always been very supportive and helpful, but he had begun to feel like he was constantly walking on eggshells due to my moodiness and irritability. He once joked, "Many evenings when I came home, I was tempted to throw my hat in the door first, and if it came flying back out I knew not to enter!"

After reading the book, I decided my next step was to find a doctor who specialized in bioidentical hormones. To my dismay, the recommended doctors listed in the back of the book were all three thousand miles away on the West Coast. My husband suggested he would buy me an airline ticket (probably one way) until I met a woman who practically saved the day—or rather saved my life! I was having a conversation with this woman, who had come to my home to install window blinds. Our conversation somehow drifted onto the subject of menopause, and I told her about the book I just read. She mentioned a friend of hers had seen a doctor in the Washington, D.C., area who had been prescribed bioidentical hormones. She stated this woman was at the point of almost selling her business due to her forgetfulness and the resulting fear of not being able to run her business anymore. After starting the bioidentical hormones, she did not sell, continued to successfully run her business, and related how she felt like she was in her thirties again! Of course, I asked my new acquaintance for this doctor's name and thus began my long relationship with Dr. Tuakli!

I must say, after the first day on the bioidentical hormones, I was amazed to wake up the next morning with the sun shining in my window! It had been three years since I had slept the night through! All my other symptoms started to diminish as well, and the best way to describe how I felt was that for the first time in years, I felt alive! My husband also said it was so nice to have his wife back!

Fast-forward to July 2012. I had been on the bioidentical hormones and feeling great for at least six years when I decided that my menopausal symptoms had been long gone and, as I approached my sixtieth birthday, that I possibly didn't need HRT anymore. I was almost at the end of my weaning-off period that fateful day in July when an unexpected and terrifying event occurred in my life. I was diagnosed with multiple sclerosis on my sixtieth birthday! I had severely diminished vision and double vision with dizziness as well as overwhelming fatigue. This would be terrifying for anyone, but being an artist, losing my sight had always been a huge fear of mine. One that came true for six weeks of my life and I hope I will never experience again.

I was diagnosed with relapsing-remitting MS. Relapsing-remitting MS is a condition in which symptoms can randomly appear (relapses) followed by partial or complete recovery (remission). My neurologist thought I had had MS for over ten years, but my relapse symptoms were vague and were misdiagnosed as something else. It took a major flare-up to be correctly diagnosed. After a week in the hospital, I was discharged with an eye patch and a walker. Gradually, six weeks later, my vision finally settled back to seminormal, and I could walk in a straight line. I had a severe reaction to the first MS drug injection I was prescribed, and my neurologist then placed me on a once-a-month infusion to slow the progression of the disease.

Over the next nine months, I was feeling a bit better but not 100 percent. Once again I started experiencing sleepless nights, and my mind began to wander back to how great I felt when I had been on the bioidentical hormones. So I picked up the phone and made an appointment with Dr. Tuakli. I was so surprised when she expressed her thoughts that removing the HRT probably caused the major MS flare up. She prescribed the bioidentical hormones, and I felt alive again!

During the next several months, everyone I encountered gushed at how wonderful I looked! And to be honest, between the bioidentical hormones and my MS infusion, I had never felt better. I never realized how bad I had been feeling over the years until I finally felt well! One day, a friend had me listen to a National Public Radio broadcast featuring one of the latest studies on MS. They believe that treating women with MS with estriol HRT diminishes flare-ups.
Needless to say, Dr. Tuakli had hit the nail on the head! Now I know why I never had a major flare-up and was able to function with my MS before I went off of my HRT. And now, with my bioidentical hormones and my MS medication, my body feels alive, and I can live everyday to the fullest!

One woman's journey.......

This is an unedited testimonial from "Songbird". She wanted me to include it in my book so others in the same special situation as her could be helped.

At 44 years old, I was diagnosed with stage IIB breast cancer. After six months of chemotherapy, along with a double mastectomy and reconstruction, I was very grateful and happy to be alive and cancer free. Then I experienced "Mr Toad's wild ride of menopause". The insomnia and hot flashes and vaginal dryness were the most obvious physical symptoms, but the mental and emotional ones were more worrisome and painful. I was forgetful and had difficulty focusing, which impacted my work performance. I suffered anxiety and low energy, resulting in a lack of self confidence. I was functioning, but it was very difficult. I tried to be positive, but I wasn't feeling the energy and zest I once had. It seemed that I was driven by sheer will and determination, but I was constantly exhausted. I went from being a vibrant, energizer bunny to a shriveled up raisin. I still worked, but it was harder to remember things and I always felt anxious. I could fall asleep at night, but could not stay asleep. I took all kinds of vitamins and sleep aids but nothing worked for any length of time. I had to muster all my strength to push myself out of bed in the morning. I was flat emotionally and became insensitive. I could watch a Nicolas Sparks movie where everyone was crying but me. I forgot to follow through on things at work and home. I had difficulty focusing to read and remembering. Sex was out of the question, as I had zero libido and was physically unable to, even if I had the desire. I thought this is as good as it gets and I would just have to accept this new kind of normal. Then one day I had a divine appointment with a wonderful doctor named Nadu Tuakli. She introduced me to bio identical hormones which I have been taking for one year. I feel like myself again. I have my emotions back. I have my passion for life back. I have my focus and memory back. No more hot flashes and anxiety. I can feel again and laugh and cry at appropriate times. I feel more energy. I can sleep for 8 hrs without waking up! I can enjoy intimacy with my husband now. What a gift. I am aging gracefully now and life is good!

NADU A. TUAKLI, MD, MPH

Differences between Compounded Hormones and Pharmaceuticals

Compounded

- always bioidentical
- pure hormone
- Biest contains 80 percent estriol
- non allergenic
- customized dose
- always bypasses the stomach

Pharmaceutical

- sometimes bioidentical
- never just pure hormone
- never contains estriol
- may cause allergies
- standard dose for everyone
- often given as a pill

Here is a poem a patient of mine wrote about the way she felt before and after BHRT.

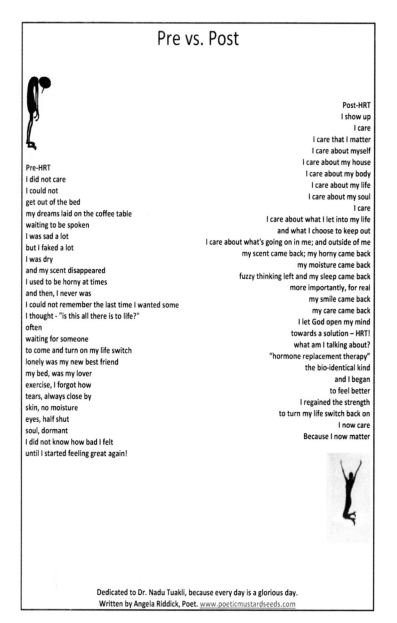

Pre vs. Post

Pre-HRT
I did not care
I could not
get out of the bed
my dreams laid on the coffee table
waiting to be spoken
I was sad a lot
but I faked a lot
I was dry
and my scent disappeared
I used to be horny at times
and then, I never was
I could not remember the last time I wanted some
I thought - "is this all there is to life?"
often
waiting for someone
to come and turn on my life switch
lonely was my new best friend
my bed, was my lover
exercise, I forgot how
tears, always close by
skin, no moisture
eyes, half shut
soul, dormant
I did not know how bad I felt
until I started feeling great again!

Post-HRT
I show up
I care
I care that I matter
I care about myself
I care about my house
I care about my body
I care about my life
I care about my soul
I care
I care about what I let into my life
and what I choose to keep out
I care about what's going on in me; and outside of me
my scent came back; my horny came back
my moisture came back
fuzzy thinking left and my sleep came back
more importantly, for real
my smile came back
my care came back
I let God open my mind
towards a solution – HRT!
what am I talking about?
"hormone replacement therapy"
the bio-identical kind
and I began
to feel better
I regained the strength
to turn my life switch back on
I now care
Because I now matter

Dedicated to Dr. Nadu Tuakli, because every day is a glorious day.
Written by Angela Riddick, Poet. www.poeticmustardseeds.com

Menopause is *always* treatable.

NADU A. TUAKLI, MD, MPH

Chapter 7

Scientific Research on Hormone Replacement Therapy

The Women's Health Initiative Study (WHI)

THERE WAS A study done in 2002 called the Women's Health Initiative. It is often referred to as the WHI study. This was a landmark study and the one that sticks in everyone's mind when they think of hormones. It is also the reason for most of the fear surrounding the use of hormones, so I am going to discuss it in great detail.

The WHI study looked at 27,347 women to study the benefits and side effects of hormone replacement in menopausal women. The study was sponsored by Wyeth, the maker of the synthetic hormones Prempro, Premarin, and Provera. At the time. Prempro (a combination of Premarin and Provera) was the second best-selling drug in the United States. Wyeth thought this study was going to show so many wonderful benefits to "hormone replacement." that people would almost want to put it in the water.

(Wyeth-Ayerst research provided the medication and placebo for the hormone study.)

Unfortunately the study backfired, and the results started to come out and were so bad the study was terminated early. Hormone therapy became maligned on the morning talk shows, and women started to throw their hormones away for fear of dying from stroke, heart attack, or breast cancer.

Sales of Prempro plummeted, at least for a while. Fortunately there were some women who were determined to find a safer hormone than completely do without, and the compounding pharmacies became extremely busy. When Wyeth realized they were losing so much of their business to the compounding pharmacies they went on the attack, and that's when suddenly there were petitions in Congress to stop compounding pharmacies, and there was a lot of noise about their products not being FDA approved.

Let's look at the WHI study and see what it taught us. Bear with me for a few pages because I'm going to get technical. It is important to understand the research when making your decision about hormones. I promise there is a light at the end of this tunnel.

The NIH (National Institutes for Health)

The NHLBI is a collaboration on the WHI study with the various parts of the NIH, including the division of Women's Health.

Here is an excerpt taken directly from the NHLBI paper about the study, from February 2010. It showed the conclusions of the first study in 2002 plus a re-analyses of the same data ten years later.

The NIH defined the WHI as a major fifteen-year research program designed to address the most frequent causes of death, disability, and poor quality of life in postmenopausal women. The study was stopped in 2002 after an average of 5.6 years of treatment due to negative findings in the women on hormones. Compared to women on placebo, women on combination hormone therapy were at increased risk of stroke, dangerous blood clots, heart disease, and breast cancer, while their risk of colorectal cancer and hip fractures was lower. So in 2002 they determined that the *overall risks of long-term use of hormone therapy outweighed the benefits.*

The study was reanalyzed by the same people ten years later and showed women who were within ten years of menopause had a *trend* toward an increased risk of heart disease, which started in the second year on the hormones. But the increased risk of heart disease *was not statistically significant.*

According to Sengwee Toh, ScD, lead author of the WHI paper and now an instructor in the Department of Population Medicine, Harvard Medical School, "This study suggests that the risk of heart disease may depend on when women start their combination hormone therapy and how long they are on this treatment." This vague statement doesn't really give us hard numbers or provide guidance as to how long after menopause starts one should begin HRT.

Jacques E. Rossouw, MD, chief of the NHLBI Women's Health Initiative branch and a coauthor of the paper, added, "Although the number of recently menopausal women who would be expected to suffer a heart attack during the first years of combination hormone therapy is *small*, the risk is likely to be real. Our findings continue to support FDA recommendations that postmenopausal hormone therapy should not be used for the prevention of heart disease."

The paper does not refer to quality-of-life issues at all.

The Cleveland Clinic

Now let's look at some of the current conclusions about the same WHI study according to the Cleveland Clinic. (Cleveland Clinic website http://my.clevelandclinic.org/health/ diseases_conditions/hic-what-is-perimenopause-menopause-postmenopause/hic_The_Womens_Health_Initiative.)

The Cleveland clinic summarizes the same WHI study, stating that only 2.5 percent of the women in this study showed negative effects. They concluded that over the course of one year, for every ten thousand women taking estrogen plus *progestin*, we would expect

- seven more women with heart attacks (as opposed to those only taking the placebo)
- eight more women with strokes
- eight more women with breast cancer
- eighteen more women with blood clots
- six fewer colorectal cancers
- five fewer hip fractures
- fewer random bone fractures

They also point out that the WHI report did not factor in the improved quality-of-life issues such as a sense of well-being, better sleep, and improvement in sexual function, skin, and hot flashes.

A positive benefit for women taking estrogen plus progestin was shown as a decrease in total cholesterol, LDL cholesterol, and triglycerides, and an increase in HDL cholesterol.

Here is my take on the WHI study:

It is generally agreed by the scientific community that the purpose of the study was to explore prevention of major chronic conditions rather than evaluating the benefit of treating symptoms. Many of the previous conclusions have been discredited over time. Clearly science is more than just numbers and many people can read the same data and come up with other conclusions. It is always possible to find research that supports diametrically opposing views but let's try and be objective here.

The WHI study made important contributions to our knowledge regarding hormone use and preventing diseases in postmenopausal women. It also challenged doctors to rethink their clinical practice. And finally it showed that synthetic hormones *at least* can have serious side effects even though they also have some positive effects.

We see that these particular hormones increase the risk of heart disease 1.29 times over the baseline risk (smoking increases your risk by 12). It is interesting to note that only those who balanced the estrogen with progestin got the benefit of decreasing colon cancer risk but lost the benefit of decreased breast cancer with estrogen alone.

But there were major problems with the WHI study: first, because Wyeth sponsored the study, only their products were used: pregnant horse estrogen (Premarin) and synthetic progestin (Provera). The information we have on BHRT has to be inferred from this data and may have nothing at all to do with it. We could be talking about apples and oranges.

We assume BHRT has the same benefits as synthetic hormones from this study, but I believe BHRT is a safer alternative because it more closely resembles what the body makes itself.

Secondly, the average age of women in the study was sixty-three, and at least 50 percent of them were reported to have had a past or current smoking history. Patients need to understand that the risks that occurred are not random events that just strike women down. They add to existing risk factors. Patients should be properly selected. Clearly a healthy woman of normal body weight who has never smoked has a different risk profile than an obese sixty-five-year-old smoker. This is before you even stratify it further based on their cholesterol levels and family history.

In the original study, there was no selectivity; no sub-analyses to tweeze out individual risk factors were performed. For instance, the seven additional women per ten thousand who would develop a myocardial infarction (heart attack) are likely to have other risk factors such as smoking, family history, high blood pressure, or increased cholesterol. We definitely know doctors need to screen who they prescribe hormones to.

Thirdly, all these products were given orally, and we know that if you swallow hormones you increase the blood-clotting factors in the liver (see chapter 6). You would anticipate an increase in blood clots, strokes, and heart attacks from this method of taking hormones because your blood gets stickier from making more clotting factors, just as it does with the oral birth-control pill. Bioidentical hormones avoid this problem.

In addition to all this, this study did not address the value of HRT for treatment of disruptive transitional symptoms, such as hot flashes and sleep disturbances, which may be a serious concern for the individual woman.

As an aside, usually only products that companies can make money from can generate the funds to sponsor large studies a big down side to objectivity.

Another recent Study

Recently (February 2015), a study came out in *Lancet* in the UK saying there may be a slight increase in the rate of ovarian cancer in HRT users. Of course this caused a lot of media attention.

Dr. Clare McKenzie, vice president of the RGOG (the Royal College of Obstetrics and Gynecology, the body that oversees OB/GYN practice in the UK), immediately said: "This study does not provide evidence that HRT is the cause of ovarian cancer ... millions of women will be confused or anxious by this 'isolated' information."

Dr. Heather Currie, chairman of the British Menopause Society, said, "Women who are currently taking HRT should not be concerned by this report. When HRT is individually tailored, it provides more benefits than risks for the majority of women under the age of sixty, and for many beyond that age."

Here is why this Lancet *study is unhelpful.* The women studied were not using bioidentical hormones. Secondly, the study was poorly done and based on only "observational data," which in science is the weakest form of data. Lastly, the supposed risk in the study was an extremely small one extra case of ovarian cancer for every thousand women on HRT, remembering that ovarian cancer itself is not a common cancer to begin with. If it encourages people to think through the kind of hormone they feel may be better and err on the side of what is more natural to the system, then that is a good thing. It would be interesting to see if the possible increase in risk of ovarian cancer from SSRI antidepressants could similarly be quantified.

Studies that Show Positive Effects of HRT

A study published in BMJ followed 1006 women age forty-five to fifty-eight for ten years, who were recently postmenopausal (average time since menopause was seven months) or had perimenopausal symptoms. Five hundred two were assigned to receive hormone-replacement therapy, and the other 504 were assigned a placebo. After ten years of follow-up, women receiving hormone-replacement therapy early after menopauses had *a significantly reduced risk of mortality, heart failure, and myocardial infarction.* This study agrees with the conclusion that beginning HRT earlier in menopause may be helpful. Remember, the women involved in this study were much younger than those in the WHI study.

There was an article in the *Lancet Oncology Journal (2012)*, which showed that after 11.8 years of follow-up from the WHI study, women who took estrogen for an average of 5.9 years actually had a *lower incidence* of invasive breast cancer (151 cases, or 0.27 percent per year compared to the placebo group: 199 cases or 0.33 percent per year).

Postgraduate Medicine is a well-known peer-reviewed journal that published a complete review article of HRT in 2009. This article reviewed all of the research available with the goal to "evaluate the evidence comparing bioidentical hormones, including progesterone, estradiol, and estriol with the commonly used non-bioidentical versions of HRT for effectiveness on symptoms, effect on breast tissue, and risks for breast cancer and cardiovascular disease."[39]

The results:

1. Patients reported greater satisfaction with HRT that contained progesterone compared to those with a synthetic progestin.
2. Bioidentical hormones have distinctly different, *potentially opposite* physiological effects than their synthetic counterparts.
3. Progesterone is associated with *diminished* risk for breast cancer compared to the synthetic progestins like Provera.
4. The negative cardiovascular (heart and arteries) effects of progestins are avoided with natural progesterone.

It concludes that "until evidence is found to the contrary, bioidentical hormones remain the preferred method of HRT. ... Research shows that bioidentical are associated with lower risks, including the risk of breast cancer and cardiovascular disease and they are more effective than the synthetic and animal derived counterparts."

So for women who prefer not to use synthetic pharmaceuticals or animal-based products in their bodies BHRT is the preferred choice on a number of levels

Estriol (E3)

One of the hormones I consider a star performer is estriol (E3), which is one of the three main estrogens we have in our bodies.

Estriol is considered the "safe" estrogen that even breast cancer survivors can take. It makes up to 80 percent of compounded Biest.

Multiple sclerosis MS is an unpredictable, often disabling disease of the central nervous system. Taking a look at the effect of estriol on MS patients can reveal just how valuable estriol is to health and well-being. In studies of MS patients in Europe, treatment with estriol proved so successful that large doses are now prescribed regularly to prevent relapses. [40]

It was observed that in pregnancy, E3 is produced in large amounts by the placenta, and since pregnant women have fewer episodes of MS, E3 was tried as a treatment. It has even been shown to significantly decrease enhancing lesions on brain MRI while the patients are on it.

Despite the fact that this form of estrogen does not cause breast cancer, it is still "not FDA approved." The FDA says its effects are not proven. Fortunately, compounding pharmacists make E3 all the time.

Hot off the press

The annual Endo conference is the most prestigious endocrinology conference in the United States and this year the 97th Annual meeting was held in San Diego, California (Endo 2015). A post-doctoral fellow at the Mayo clinic Khalid Benkhadra MD and his colleagues presented a paper at Endo 2015 showing a meta-analysis of 43 randomized trials about HRT including WHI. The study included over 52,000 women with a mean age of 62 and average follow up of 5 years on HRT and their conclusion was that HRT did *not* affect women's mortality one way or the other. There was no significant association between HRT use and all cause mortality, or mortality due to heart attack, breast cancer or stroke. The results were similar for estrogen only and combination therapy.

So HRT neither negatively nor positively impacted mortality. This is huge, bye-bye rumors! [44]

What about the cost? Is It Worth It?

UK Menopausal Study

Another study done 2009 [46] in the UK explored whether treatment of menopause was a cost-effective strategy—in other words, did it work well enough for the health care system to be reimbursing it.

In England, more than 90 percent of the people are covered by the National Healthcare System (NHS), which is run by the government. The study looked at clinical effects of HRT on: Hip fractures, vertebral fractures, wrist fractures, breast cancer, colon cancer, coronary heart disease, stroke and venous thromboembolic events (blood clots).

The researchers compared the quality-adjusted life year (QALY) gained from HRT to that with no treatment. The study concluded in the affirmative: HRT is worth spending money on. It *was* cost effective for the NHS to treat women with menopausal symptoms with HRT.

The severity of menopausal symptoms was the single most important determinant of cost effectiveness, but they found that HRT was "still cost effective even where symptoms were mild or effects on symptom relief were small."

Conclusion: treatment of women with menopausal symptoms with HRT is worth it.

I think in the US the insurance companies could learn something from this study, women should demand their hormone prescriptions be covered.

Stay active

Other studies have shown that increasing body fat is related to increasing risk of uterine cancer. it is also a factor in the development of breast, colon and possibly ovarian cancer. Some scientists believe that one-third of cancer deaths in women are due to excess body weight.

There is definitely a well-known link between exercise and breast cancer. Epidemiologic studies have shown that breast cancer risk is reduced by 30 to 40 percent in highly active females compared to inactive women.

Summary

So to summarize from this overview of selective scientific studies:

Studies show that treating menopause is effective and worth the money. Some show that in younger menopausal women there is a reduction in heart disease and possibly decreased breast cancer if progesterone is used. BHRT is safer, more effective, and distinctly different physiologically compared to synthetic hormones.

Exercise is good for everyone and has been shown to prevent cancer [47, 48, 49, 50].

> "Over-interpretation and misrepresentation of the WHI findings have damaged the health and well-being of menopausal women by convincing them and their health professionals that the risks of HT outweigh the benefits"[45]

Chapter 8

Are Hormones Right for Me?

Where Do You Find Help?

Choosing Your Doctor

Can you guide your doctor?

A CTUALLY, YOU MAY *have* to, which is why you need to be informed.

Every woman deserves the right to personalized care. If you think your doctor is not hearing your concerns or is too busy to address them, find someone else. A doctor needs to be knowledgeable and willing to work with you to find the best customized solution for you. You may need to try a variety of compounds over time before you find one that works for you as your circumstances change.

Most medical doctors have received no training whatsoever in menopause, and this includes gynecologists. Students in medical school don't even get one full lecture on the subject.

A lot of people assume that because BHRT is a "woman's issue," the place to go is to a gynecologist's office. But unless a GYN has had special training in the subject, they are unfamiliar with BHRT. Since most of the symptoms of menopause are above the belly button, a gynecologist may actually not be the kind of doctor you are looking for anyway.

In the online journal *Menopause* [51] published in the fall of 2013 a survey of all OB/GYN residency programs showed that fewer than 20 percent of resident GYN doctors had received any formal training in menopause. According to the author of the study new residents readily admitted that their knowledge and clinical management skills of menopause were inadequate. More than 70 indicated that they were not trained to handle menopause and did not feel confident doing so.

In a 2014 article in the Johns Hopkins monthly medical magazine, a female professor expressed concerns about how many women with menopausal symptoms were being given Valium and Xanax and then ended up being drug-dependent later in life. She suggested lack of training and the doctor's prescribing habits were increasing the rates of drug addiction in the community.

One could argue that the risks of these tranquilizers as well as sleeping medications outweigh the potential risk of hormone therapy.

Even though menopause involves hormones, do not expect an endocrinologist to be particularly helpful with this kind of hormone replacement, as very few are familiar with BHRT.

In fact, there is no specific "specialty" that indicates which doctor will be well-versed in BHRT. That is because specializing in menopause is motivated by a physician's specific interest in the subject. That interest is what drives the physician to seek out information and attend courses on her own. The doctor must then acquire experience through practice. There are very few role models for young doctors and no formal apprenticeships.

A paper was written in the Journal of Women's Health in April 2014 calling for more internists to be trained in menopause management. The authors wrote that "Most internists currently lack the core competencies and experience necessary to address menopausal issues and meet the needs of women who have completed their reproductive years." [52, 53] The conclusion of the paper was a proposal that "the multidimensional expertise" that characterizes (Primary Care) would provide the most comphrehensive approach to menopause management. They also suggested that new didactic programs be developed for medical students, residents and practicing physicians. It is unfortunate, that articles still need to be written to suggest this in 2014!

One type of BHRT does not work for everyone, so therapy has to be tailored for each individual patient. The therapy is adjusted according to their hormone levels which should be monitored. I always use the lowest combination "enough to do the job but no more than you need." Remember that every woman has a unique response to a particular dose, hormone combination and mode of delivery.

If you are seeking a BHRT physician in your area, here are two avenues to try.

Almost all doctors who refer to themselves as "anti-aging" physicians are quite familiar with the art of bioidentical hormones. Seminars they attend offer bioidentical hormones as a prominent topic of discussion. I personally enjoy these gatherings because it is nice to exchange ideas with like-minded physicians, and there are thousands of them. They come from the full spectrum of medical specialties, and they are all seeking better ways to help women optimize their health. You can do an internet search for this kind of doctor.

The second thing you could do would be to call a reputable compounding pharmacy (see discussion below) and ask for references.

Once you have chosen a doctor and fully researched his or her background, make an appointment for an initial consultation. This way you can interview the doctor and have your questions answered without making a commitment. Ask questions like, "How can I determine my P/E (progesterone/estrogen) ratio?" If the doctor asks, "What's that?" you are probably in the wrong place.

At the first visit the doctor will want to know:

- If you smoke
- If you have had any cancer
- Your family history
- If you or a family member has ever had blood clots in the veins
- If you have any gallbladder or liver disease
- Any history of heart disease
- Your family history of osteoporosis

Depending on your responses and your age hormone therapy may or may not be for you. Everything has to be put in perspective and this requires you and your physician to evaluate your individual risk-benefit assessment.

What is a Compounding Pharmacy?

You can *only* get combination bioidentical hormones at a compounding pharmacy. Towards the back of the book I have included a resource section where I have put the contact information for some of the pharmacies that we use. Even if you are not ready to start hormones the compounding pharmacists are great resources. The are always willing to answer your questions and send you additional informational material if necessary. One other great thing about compounding pharmacies is that most of them will mail you your prescription. Depending on where they are licensed, they will ship to other states as well.

Most people do not realize a compounding pharmacist is specially trained and has chosen to do extra training above and beyond regular pharmacy school. This allows them to create customized prescriptions. Scaremongers would have you believe you are getting an inferior product if it doesn't come in standard one-size-fits-all type of pills.

Traditional doctors love to say that they are not regulated. What hogwash! Can you imagine people being allowed to dispense medications in the United States with no oversight? And then there is the comment about not being FDA approved. This is true. Of course the traditional experts are basing that comment on a technicality: each individual compound is not specifically FDA approved because it's made for the specific consumer. Estriol as a compound has not been FDA approved *not* because of side effects but because they say it hasn't been proven to be effective (see chapter 7).

Remember "its not FDA approved" is not synonymous with "its dangerous". Millions of physicians use medications for non FDA approved indications daily.

One of the things I like best is that bioidentical hormones are compounded with the exact amount that is prescribed for a specific patient. If I want my patient to have 0.55 mg. of a hormone, that is exactly what they get, not 0.50 mg.

One thing that you never hear from a compounding pharmacist is, "It doesn't come in that size."

As with everything else these days you can check your pharmacy's track record and regulation compliance status online. Do not be concerned about hype and rumors.

An Accountant Trying to Keep the Numbers Straight

Ten years ago, when "Maggie N." was fifty, she came to see me, and she was definitely ahead of the curve. Two years prior she had had a total abdominal hysterectomy and both ovaries removed (TAHBSO) for fibroid tumors in the uterus. Apart from lactose intolerance and a little hypoglycemia she was otherwise healthy. She had always maintained a healthy weight, although recently it had started creeping up. She was 146 pounds and 66 inches tall with a BMI of 23.6.

She was distressed by her decreased memory, and it had gotten particularly bad over the past year. She had been put on an estradiol patch after her hysterectomy, which made her edgy and itchy, then she was switched to another one which seemed to make her hair fall out. "I have no libido and my husband is going crazy," she said.

Two years after starting on her BHRT, Maggie was feeling great! So good in fact that she decided that any doctor could prescribe her hormones and she asked her gynecologist to take over prescribing them. We didn't see her for sixteen months. As her symptoms changed, her doctor would adjust her prescription, and she would feel worse. She had continued to get her prescription at the same pharmacy and would complain to the pharmacist, who finally told her what she had already figured out: "You need to go back; not everyone specializes in hormones."

"Can I come back? My 'regular' doctor means well, but she ain't no Dr. T!" she told my office manager.

Maggie had become very moody and edgy again. She was having headaches, which she rated as 6 out of 10, was depressed (5 out of 10), her breasts were very tender, and her overall well-being was now up to 7 out of 10 (from 3). We had to go back to the drawing board with a complete reevaluation, I found she was completely out of balance. Happily she is now 10 years later she is well balanced (see her chart from 2014 below). She now weighs 125 pounds and does Zumba three days a week. Her memory is 100 percent back to normal, clearly a critical issue for an accountant.

Every time she comes in she smiles radiantly and says "I feel better than I did at 35 and my husband agrees completely!"

Symptom profile for Maggie
"Keeping the numbers straight"

SYMPTOM	Start	One month on BHRT	Six months	Prior to leaving	✱ 4 years later on return	7 years later	10 years later (now)
Fatigue	7	2	4	3	6	3	2
Quality of sleep	6	2	3	2	7	4	3
Energy	7	2	3	3	7	3	2
Libido	9	2	3	2	6	3	3
Weight	5	2	4	4	3	5	2
Exercise	4	2	2	2	4	2	1
Headaches	4	5	4	3	8	2	2
Skin	5	3	3	2	2	3	3
Depression	1	1	1	1	5	1	1
Mood swings	1	1	1	1	7	1	1
Memory	9	7	5	3	3	1	1
Overall well being	5	3	3	3	7	2	2

**the patient was getting her prescription elsewhere

NADU A. TUAKLI, MD, MPH

Chapter 9

Interesting Facts about Women's Health

S OME OF THIS information has been discussed in the book but is worth mentioning again, and some not related to hormone balancing is still information women should be aware of.

Life Expectancy

One hundred years ago women were not expected to live much past forty-eight. Today the average life expectancy for women in the United States is eighty-one.

Heart Disease

Heart disease is the number-one cause of death in women in the United States (23.5%).

Cancer is second (22.1%) and stroke third (6.2%). [55]

Cancer Risk

Losing weight reduces cancer risk. The loss of 5 percent body weight in an obese woman reduces her risk of cancer by 50 percent. [47, 48, 49]

The top 3 cancer deaths in women (2014 data) were: [56]

1. Respiratory system cancers (73,380)
2. All Digestive system cancers (62,290)
3. Breast (40,000)

Breast cancer

Risk factors associated with a higher incidence of breast cancer include

- Race: Caucasians have a higher incidence than African American and Asian women.
- starting periods before age twelve and menopause after fifty-five
- having first child after thirty
- radiation to the chest more than ten years before
- denser breasts
- smoking
- Women who drink alcohol have a higher incidence than those who don't
- higher BMI (overweight/obesity)
- Studies have shown that breast cancer risk is reduced by 30 to 40 percent in highly physically active women when compared with inactive ones.[3]
- BRCA mutations are related to a 3 to 4 percent increase risk of breast cancer but the proportion of ovarian cancer due to BRCA is much higher, the increased ovarian cancer risk is 15 percent [57,58]

Tubal Ligation

Tubal ligation can change your periods and bring menopause on earlier. Most women complain of increased flow and sometimes more cramping. On the other hand, women who have had a tubal ligation have a lower incidence of ovarian cancer. It is thought that ovarian cancer actually starts in the fallopian tubes. I believe that is why it seems to come on

---

[3] Peplonska B, Lissowska J, et al. Adulthood lifetime physical activity and breast cancer, *Epidemiology*. 2008 Mar;19(2):226-36. doi: 10.1097/EDE.0b013e3181633bfb.

so suddenly. By the time it gets to the ovaries, you are dealing with a cancer that is already spreading, whereas when it is in the tubes you can't see or feel it. [59, 60, 61]

Hysterectomy

More than half a million hysterectomies are performed in the United States annually. The average age for the procedure is forty. Only 10.7 percent are for cancerous conditions. If the ovaries are removed before sixty-five, a woman's risk of death from all causes is increased. Hysterectomy may be associated with weight gain.

Fibroids

By age fifty, 70 percent of white women and 80 percent of African Americans have fibroids. Most fibroids are harmless, but when they are big they can cause pressure symptoms and interfere with pregnancy. It is unusual for them to be the cause of uncontrollable bleeding by themselves.

The least invasive way to get rid of them is by embolization of the uterine artery, dietary changes will not make your fibroids shrink.

Alzheimer's

Some studies have shown that synthetic hormones increase the risk of dementia [63]. According to the Alzheimer's Foundation of America, five million people suffer from Alzheimer's and the incidence is rising. Two-thirds of Americans with Alzheimer's are women. The incidence doubles every five years after age sixty-five.

It is estimated that in the next forty years the number of cases will triple.

Osteoporosis

Women who use Depo-Provera Contraceptive Injection may lose significant bone mineral density resulting in osteoporosis. Depo-Provera is medroxyprogesterone, also known as Provera. [64, 65]

Osteoporosis is the fourth leading cause of death in women, following heart disease, cancer, and stroke. Death from osteoporosis is usually a result of complications that follow bone fractures.

One and a half million fractures occur from osteoporosis annually in the United States, resulting in 2.6 million doctor visits and 300,000 hospitalizations.

Twenty-four percent of the 300,000 people who sustain hip fractures die within a year.

The surgeon general's office report on the subject stated that by the year 2020, half of all Americans older than fifty would be at risk for fractures from osteoporosis. Of women who are currently fifty or older, 40 percent will suffer a fracture of the hip, wrist, or spine at some point in their lives. The same report points out that nine out of ten teenage girls do not get enough calcium.

By age eighty, smokers have 6 to 10 percent lower bone density than nonsmokers.

Depression

A woman who has had post partum depression is at higher risk for depression during perimenopause and menopause.

Resources

Dr. Nadu Tuakli MD, MPH

10814 Hickory ridge Road
Columbia, MD 21044

410 992 0011

www.anti-agingdoctor.com

Professional Arts Pharmacy

2015 Lord Baltimore Drive
Baltimore, MD 21244

443-200-1200
1-800-832-9285
443 200-1209 (fax)

Email: Sam@WeMakeMeds.com

www.WeMakeMeds.com

Voshell's Pharmacy

3455 Wilkens Ave
Baltimore, MD 21229

410 644 8400
410 368 5110 (fax)

Pharmacist: Jay Dorsch

www.voshellspharmacy.com

Chambers' Apothecary

278 Lincoln Way East
Chambersburg, PA 17201

717 263 0747
1 844 256 7025
717 263 0225 (fax)

Email: info@chambersapothecary.com

www.chambersapothecary.com

References

Intro

1. Preamble to the constitution of the World Health organization (see foot note on page one)

Chapter One

2. Could transdermal estradiol +progesterone be a safer postmenopausal HRT? A review.
   L'hermite M; Simoncini T; Fuller S; Genazzani AR.
   Mauritas. 60 (3-4): 185-201, 2008 Jul-Aug.

3. HRT optimization, using transdermal estradiol plus micronized progesterone, a safer HRT (Review).
   L'Hermite M.
   Climacteric. 16 Suppl 1:44-53, 2013 Aug.

4. Differential effects of oral and transdermal postmenopausal estrogen replacement therapies on C-reactive protein.
   Lacut K; Le Gal G; et al.
   Thrombosis and haemostasis. 90 (1):124-31, 2003 Jul.

5. Attitude of German women towards hormone therapy: results of a lay survey.
   Buhling KJ; Daniels Bet al.
   Gynecological Endocrinology. 29(5):460-4, 2013 May.

6. A multicentric study regarding the use of hormone therapy during female mid-age
   Blumel JE: Chedraui P, Baron G; et al.
   Climacteric. 17(4):433-41,2014 Aug.

Symptoms

7. Risk of long-term hot flashes after natural menopause: evidence from the Penn Ovarian Aging Study cohort.
   Freeman EW; Sammel MD; Sanders RJ.
   Menopause. 21(9): 924-32, 2014 Sep. (journal article)

8. Factors associated with reporting classic menopausal symptoms differ.
   Duffy OK; Iversen L; Hannford PC.
   Climacteric. 16(2):240-51, 2013 Apr.

9. Menopausal hormonal therapy and menopausal symptoms(Review Journal Article)
   Al-safi ZA; Santoro N.
   Fertility and Sterility. 101(4):905-15, 2014 Apr

10. Age of menopause and impact of climacteric symptoms by geographical region.
    Palacios S;Henderson VW; Siseles N; Tan D; Villaseca P.
    Climacteric. 13(5): 419-28, 2010 Oct.

11. The impact of menopausal symptoms on work ability.
    Geukes M; van Aalst MP; Nauta MC; Oosterhof H.
    Menopause. 19(3):278-82, 2012 Mar.

12. Gender and the effects of steroid hormones in the central nervous system
    Brandt N;Vierk R; Fester L; Zhou L; Imholz P; Rune GM
    Bundesgesundheitsblatt, Gesundheitsforschung, Geshundheitsschutz. 57(9): 1054-1060 2014 Sep.

13. Hormone replacement therapy- is there a place for its use in neurology?
    Vukovic V; Lovrencic-Huzjan A; Solter VV et al.
    Ollegium Antropologicum. 27(1): 413-24,2003 Jun

14. Hormone sensitive seizure in women with epilepsy
    Shafer, PO.
    Clinical Nursing practice in Epilesy. 4(3):8-10, 1997

15. Menopausal symptoms appear before the menopause and persist 5 years

beyond: a detailed analysis of a multinational study.
Blumel JE; Chedraui P; Baron G et al.
Climacteric. 15(6):542-51, 2012 Dec.

16. Frequency of symptoms and health seeking behaviours of menopausal women in an out-patient clinic in Port Harcourt, Nigeria.
Dienye PO; Judah F; Ndukwu G.
Global Journal of Health Science. 5(4):39-47, 2013 Jul.

17. Experience of menopausal symptoms by women in an urban community in Ibadan, Nigeria
Olalorun FM; Lawoyin TO
Menopause. 16(4):822-30, 2009 Jul-Aug

18. Severe menopausal symptoms in mid-aged Latin American women can be related to their indigenous ethnic component
E. Ojeda, A. monterrosa, J.E Blumel, J. Escobar-Lopez and P. Chedraui
Climacteric 2011;14:157-13

19. http:www.cdc.gov/women/lcod/2010/womenrace_2010.pdf

20. The relationship between urogenital symptoms and climacteric complaints
Oge T; Hassa H; Aydin Y; et al.
Climacteric. 16(6):646-52, 2013 Dec.

21. (Mood disorders in perimenopausal women: hormone replacement or antidepressant therapy?). (Review) (27 refs) English abstract
Bertschy G; de Ziegler D; Bianchi-Demicheli F.
Revue medicale Suisse. 1 (330:2155-6, 2159-61, 2005 Sep 21

22. Hot flushes still occur in a population of 85-year-old Swedish women.
Vikstrom, J; Spetz Holm, A-C et al.
Climacteric. 16(4): 453-9, 2013 Aug.

Sexual Intimacy

23. Association between Higher Levels of Sexual Function, Activity, and Satisfaction and Self-Rated Successful Aging in Older Postenopausal Women.

Wesley Thompson, PhD, et al.
J Am Geriatr Soc. August 2011; 59(8): 1503-1508. Published online July 28,2011.
Doi:10.1111/j.1532-5415.2011.03495.x.

24. A prospective cohort study on the effect of sexual activity, libido and widowhood on mortality among elderly people: 14 year follow-up of 2453 elderly Taiwanese.
Chen JK, Tseng CD, Wu SC, Lee TK et al.
The International Journal of Epidemiology. 36(5):1136-42

25. Sex and Death: are they related? Findings from the Caerphilly cohort study. *BMJ:*315: 1641

26. Menopause negatively impacts sexual lives of middle-aged Iranian women: a cross-sectional study
Mergati-Khoei E, Sheikhan F; Shamsalizadeh N; Haghani H; et al.
Journal of Sex and Marital Therapy. 40(6):552-60, 2014.

Treatment

27. A controlled trial of intravaginal estriol in postmenopausal women with recurrent urinary tract infections.
Raz R; Stamm WE.
New England Journal of Medicine. 329(11):753-6, 1993 Sep 9.

28. Estriol in the management of the menopause
Tzingounis VA; Aksu MF; Greenblatt RB.
JAMA. 239 (16):1638-41, 1978 Apr 21

29. Estriol:safety and efficacy.
Head KA.
Alternative Medicine Review. 3(2):101-13, 1998 Apr.

30. Vaginal atrophy in breast cancer survivors: role of vaginal estrogen therapy.
Mariani L; Gadducci A; Vizza E et al.
Gynecological Endocrinology. 29(1)25-9, 2013 Jan.

NADU A. TUAKLI, MD, MPH

31. Efficacy and safety of oral estriol for managing postmenopausal symptoms.
Takahashi K; Manabe A et al.
Maturitas. 34(2): 169-77, 2000 Feb 15.

32. Efficacy and safety of estriol replacement therapy for climacteric women.
Yang TS; Tsan SH et al.
Chung Hua I Hsueh Tsa Chih - Chinese Medical Journal 55(5): 386-91, 1995 May

33. Estriol (E3) replacement improves endothelial function and bone mineral density in very elderly women.
Hyashi T; Ito l; Kano H et al.

34. *Journals of Gerontology Series A- Biological Sciences & Medical Sciences. 55(4):B183-90 200 Apr.*
(Breast cancer risk is increased for patients on estradiol only)

35. Breast cancer risk in postmenopausal women using estrogen-only therapy.
Lyythinen, Heli; Pukkala, Eero et al.
Obstetrics and gynecology. 108(6):1354-60, 2006 Dec

36. Effects of estriol on the proliferation and differentiation of human osteoblastic MG-63 cells.
Luo XH; Liao EY.
Endocrine research. 29(3): 343-51, 2003 Aug.

37. Hormone replacement containing progestins and given continuously increases breast cancer risk in Sweden
Olsson HL; Ingvar C; Bladstrom A.
Cancer. 97(6):1387-92, 2003 Mar 15.

38. The effects of compounded bioidentical transdermal hormone therapy on hemostatic, inflammatory, imue factors; cardiovascular biomarkers; quality-of-life measures; and health outcomes in perimenopausal and post menopausal women.
Stephenson K; Neuenschwander PF et al.

International Journal of Pharmaceutical Compound. 17(1): 74-85, 2013 Jan-Feb.

39. The bioidentical hormone debate: are bioidentical hormones (estradiol, estriol, and progesterone) safer or more efficacious than commonly used synthetic versions in hormone replacement therapy?
Holtorf K.
Postgraduate Medicine. 121(1):73-85, 2009 Jan. (Review of articles)

Research

40. Immune modulation in multiple sclerosis patients treated with the preganacy hormone Estriol.
Soldan SS; Alvarez Retuerto Al; Sicotte NL et al.
Journla of immunology. 17(11):6267-74, 2003 Dec 1.

41. Review of clinical trial where estriol and testosterone showed a shift from a pro-inflammatory state to an anti-inflammatory state.
Haldane J.
J Orthomol Med. 2012; 27:87-92

42. Does hormone replacement therapy cause breast cancer? An application of causal principles to three studies. Part 4: the million women study.
Shapiro S; Farmer Rd et al.
Journal of Family Planning and Reproductive Health Care. 38(2):102-9, 20012 Apr.

43. What if the Womens Health Initiative had used transdermal estradiol and progesterone instead?
Simon, James A.
Menopause. 21(7):769-83,2014 Jul.

44. *The Endocrine Society annual meeting. ENDO 2015 Abstract FRI-125, presented March 6 2015. Khalid Benkhadra et al.*

45. Risks and benefits of hormone therapy: has medical dogma now been overturned?
Shapiro S; de Viliers TJ; Pines A et al.
Climecteric. 17(3):215-22,2014 Jun

46. Cost-effectiveness of hormone replacement therapy for menopausal symptoms in the UK
Ingrid Lekander, Frederik Borgstrom et al.
Menopause International 2009; *15: 19-25. DOI: 10.1258/mi.2009.009004*

47. Effects of aerobic training on menopausal symptoms- a randomized trial
Moilanen JM; Mikkola TS; Raitanen JA et al
Menopause. 19(6): 691-6, 2012 Jun.
(n=176 age 45 to 63)

48. Body mass index, physical activity, and mortality in women diagnosed with ovarian cancer: results from the Women's Health Initiative.
Zhou Y; Chlebowski R; Lamonte MJ et al.
Gynecologic Oncology. 133 (1):4-10, 2014 Apr.

49. Adulthood lifetime physical activity and breast cancer.
Peplonska B, Lissowska J et al.
Epidemiology 2008 Mar: 19(2) :226-36.doi:10.1097/EDE.ObO13e3181633bfb.

50. The risk of uterine malignancy is linearly associated with the body mass index in a cohort of US women.
Ward KK, Roncancio AM, Shah NR et al.
AM J Obstet Gynecol. 2013 Dec;209(6):579.e 1-5.doi:

Medical Providers

51. Menopause education: needs assessment of American obstetrics and gynecology residents.
Christianson MS; Ducie JA; Altmen K et al.
Menopause. 20(11):1120-5, 2013 Nov.

52. Competency in menopause management: whither goes the internist?
Santen RJ; Stuenkel CA; Burger HG et al.
Journal of Women's Health. 23(4):281-5, 2014 Apr

53. Focused teaching in menopause: the time is now
Berkowitz LR.
Menopause. 19(10):1072-3, 2012 Oct

54. Working women and menopause
Menopause and work—the experience of middle-aged female teaching staff in an Egyptian governmental faculty of medicine.
Hammam RA; Abbas RA; Hunter MS.
Mauritas. 71(3):294-300, 2012 Mar.

Interesting Facts

55. www.cdc.gov/women/lcod/2010/WomenRace_2010.pdf

56. Top 3 cancer deaths in women (2014 data)
Siegel R, Ma J et al.
Cancer statistics, 2014 CA: A Cancer Journal for Clinicians.
64(1): 9-29. DOI: 10.3322/caac.21208

57. Realizing the promise of cancer predisposition.
Rahman N.
Nature. 2014;505:302-308

58. Article: 20 years since BRCA: where are we now in cancer screening?
Medscape. Apr 13, 2015

59. Incidence of Ovarian Cancer with Tubal Ligation:
Tubal ligation, Hystrectomy, unilateral oophorectomy and risk of ovarian cancer in the Nurses health Studies.
Rice MS, Hankinson SE, and Tworoger SS (2014)
Fertility and Sterility. 102(1): 192-198

60. Tubal sterilization and risk of ovarian, endometrial and cervical cancer.
Kjaer SK, Mellemkjaer L et al.
International Journal of Epidemiology. 33930:596-602.

61. Mathematical models of ovarian cancer incidence
Rosner BA, Colditz GA, et al.
Epidemiology. 16(4):508-15.

62. Is maternal height a risk factor for breast cancer?
Lagiou P; Trichopoulos D; Hsieh CC

European Journal of cancer prevention. 22(5):389-90, 2013 Sep
(taller mothers positively associated with birth size and breast cancer risk

63. Combination hormone replacement therapy and dementia.
Wooltorton E
Canadian medical Association Journal. 169(2):133,2003 Jul 22

64. Medroxyprogesterone acetate (Depo-Provera) and bone mineral density loss.
Wooltorton E.
CMJ Canadian Medical Association Journal. 172(6):746, 2005 Mar 15

65. The FDA, contraceptive marketing approval and products liability litigation: Depo-Provera and the risk of osteoporosis.
Green W.

Index

hot flashes (flushes), 3, 29, 34, 38–39, 42–43, 48, 50, 53, 62–63, 71, 74–75, 82–83, 87, 90, 96–97

hysterectomy, 11, 14, 32, 44, 107, 111

I

incontinence, 51

insomnia, 26, 31, 38, 40, 43, 73, 90

interstitial cystitis, 51, 61

J

joint pain, 23, 38, 74

L

LH, 17

libido, 22–23, 50, 56–60, 69, 71–72, 75, 80–81, 83, 87, 90, 107

lock and key mechanism, 15

M

melatonin, 14, 48

menopause myths, 11

mood swings, 40, 46–47, 71, 83

multiple sclerosis, 19, 40, 49, 88, 100

O

osteoporosis, 22, 24, 41, 50, 74, 80, 85, 105, 112

P

palpitations, 27, 41, 51

perimenopause, 17, 22–23, 25–26, 28–32, 35–36, 45, 47–48, 50–51, 53, 55, 57, 65, 67–69, 85, 95

physicians/doctors, 3–5, 9–11, 22, 25–28, 30, 32, 36, 48–50, 52, 61–62, 78–79, 85–86, 88, 96–97, 103–7

PMS, 21, 24, 35–36, 47–48, 85

pregnenolone, 16, 20

Premarin, 19–20, 76, 93, 96

Prempro, 20, 93

progesterone, 8, 14, 16–18, 20–22, 24, 28, 30, 33–34, 57, 60, 74, 76–77, 79–81, 86, 99

progestin, 20, 95–96, 99

Provera, 20–21, 74, 76, 80, 93, 96, 99, 112

S

saliva testing, 22

serotonin, 46, 48, 69, 72–73

sexual dysfunction, 17, 57, 61–62, 81

T

testosterone, 4, 6, 8, 14, 16–17, 19, 22, 33, 57, 60, 77, 80–81, 84, 86

V

vaginal dryness, 10, 38, 40, 44, 61–62, 80, 90

W

weight gain, 23, 39, 44–45, 72, 111

Women's Health Initiative Study (WHI), 20, 80, 93

X

Xanax, 45, 72, 104

NADU A. TUAKLI, MD, MPH